PSEUDOMONAS
AERUGINOSA

Pseudomonas Aeruginosa: Ecological Aspects and Patient Colonization

Edited by

Viola Mae Young, Ph.D.

Head, Microbiology Section
Baltimore Cancer Research Center
National Cancer Institute
Baltimore, Maryland

Raven Press ■ New York

Raven Press, 1140 Avenue of the Americas, New York, New York 10036

Library of Congress Cataloging in Publication Data

Main Entry under title:

Pseudomonas aeruginosa: ecological aspects and patient colonization

Includes bibliographies and index.

I. Pseudomonas disease --Congresses. 2. Pseudomonas aeruginosa--Congresses. 3. Nosocomial infections--Congresses. 4. Epidemiology--Congresses. 5. Microbial-ecology--Congresses. I. Young, Viola Mae. II. American Society for Microbiology
RC II6.P7P73   6I6.9'2   76-569I9
ISBN 0-89004-I49-0

Preface

My aim in organizing this publication is to cross the unnatural barriers that exist between various disciplines and to bring together the information essential to the understanding of the single microorganism *P. aeruginosa*. In our education and in our experience, we are too frequently limited or fenced, as it were, by the boundaries of a profession or a discipline. Such boundaries may be necessary; they obviously serve a useful purpose. But a microorganism need not necessarily respect such limits. The ecological niche of an organism such as *P. aeruginosa* is indeed complex, and a clear understanding of its ecology as well as appreciation of its versatility would involve knowledge in the disciplines of microbiology (plant and animal,) plant pathology, sanitation, environmental health, and others. By crossing the barriers of these disciplines, the knowledge essential to understanding is brought together and the first steps toward control of *P. aeruginosa* and prevention of its acquisition by hospitalized patients can be made.

This organism, which is an "opportunistic" pathogen in both plants and animals, obviously has a number of tricks up its genetic sleeve, but these are not dealt with here. Rather, we have tried to show where *P. aeruginosa* is found in nature, indicated some areas of its importance in that natural environment, documented some of the means by which it reaches the hospital environment and some of the sites within the hospital that it may colonize. From there it is a short step to the patient where it constitutes a serious threat if host defenses are damaged so that the patient is left at high risk of infection. It is imperative for the scientist to "know the enemy." Armed with knowledge of the factors that contribute to patient colonization and infection, one can validly interfere with such an eventuality.

I gratefully acknowledge the enthusiastic support given by the excellent scientists, who have such varied backgrounds, but who were united in their common interest in an unusual organism; this interest led to their participation and to their preparation of manuscripts for this book. The constant cooperation of my associate, Ms. Marcia R. Moody, is also enormously helpful. Lastly, I wish to express gratitude to my secretary, Ms. Judy Schuler, whose understanding and dedication are invaluable.

Viola Mae Young

Contents

Contributors

John J. Cho
Department of Plant Pathology
University of California
Berkeley, California 94720

Charles E. Copeland
Division of General Surgery
Mercy Hospital
Pittsburgh, Pennsylvania 15219

Carol A. Delenko
Division of General Surgery
Mercy Hospital
Pittsburgh, Pennsylvania 15219

Sylvia K. Green
Department of Plant Pathology
University of California
Berkeley, California 94720

Alfred W. Hoadley
School of Civil Engineering
Georgia Institute of Technology
Atlanta, Georgia 30332

Ian Alan Holder
Shriner's Burns Institute
Departments of Microbiology and
  Surgery
University of Cincinnati College of
  Medicine
Cincinnati, Ohio 45219

Spyros Kominos
Microbiology Section
Mercy Hospital
Pittsburgh, Pennsylvania 15219

Matthew E. Levison
Division of Infectious Diseases,
  Allergy and Immunology
The Medical College of
  Pennsylvania
Philadelphia, Pennsylvania 19129

Marcia R. Moody
Baltimore Cancer Research Center
National Cancer Institute
Baltimore, Maryland 21201

Milton N. Schroth
Department of Plant Pathology
University of California
Berkeley, California 94720

Introduction

It is not always appreciated that *Pseudomonas aeruginosa* is an ubiquitous organism, able to flourish in multiple environments, possibly enabled to do so by its ability to utilize many different organic compounds as energy sources and to survive for lengthy periods as long as sufficient moisture is available. Also, it is not uncommon to recover *P. aeruginosa* from humans. A small, but definite, percentage (3% to approximately 19%) of normal individuals have been shown to carry *P. aeruginosa* in their gastrointestinal tracts. In my own observations of the fecal flora of 5 nonhospitalized normal individuals over a 6-month period *(unpublished data),* episodes of loose stools or diarrhea were most frequently followed by transient recovery of this organism. The ways by which *P. aeruginosa* is introduced to man are varied; it is likely that many normal adults have frequent contact with this organism either from the food they eat, the water they drink, the water from faucets colonized with *P. aeruginosa* in which they bathe, the water in pools where they swim, or the plants with which they decorate their homes. Some investigators, including Hoadley, believe it probable that this bacterium is primarily associated with man, whereas others believe it possible that "soil and plants serve as natural and permanent reservoirs for the bacterium" (Schroth et al.).

Indeed, the genus *Pseudomonas* encompasses a great number of species that are phytopathogenic. Historically, over 220 names for these phytopathogens have been published in the genus *Pseudomonas* Migula, 1894, although some are considered to be invalid or illegitimate for various reasons, such as inadequate original descriptions, invalid publication, and so forth. These problems were understandable as the techniques that were available to the earlier investigators did not allow precise species differentiation of this genus. As newer techniques became available, it became possible to identify *P. aeruginosa* with some certainty. By 1942, Elrod and Braun reported that one of the pseudomonads capable of causing a pathogenic process in plants, *P. polycolor,* was identical to *P. aeruginosa.*

Subspeciation of this organism by means of serotyping, bacteriophage typing, and pyocin typing has further enabled investigators to trace this organism through the multiple environments in which it flourishes. Thus, Kominos et al. were able to demonstrate that many of the pyocin types of *P. aeruginosa* that were found in samples from vegetables were the same as those recovered from patients, indicating that both plants and humans could serve as hosts for the same strains of *P. aeruginosa.* Moody *(unpublished data)* utilized serotyping to test strains of *P. aeruginosa* recovered from vegetables and humans and came to a similar conclusion.

Nevertheless, problems in differentiation of the pseudomonads, particularly the fluorescent species, still exist and do not lend themselves readily to simple solutions by the uninitiated. Furthermore, the considerable frequency with which nonpigmented strains of *P. aeruginosa* are recovered in botanical, clinical, and environmental microbiology laboratories makes it essential to employ optimal techniques in differentiating these strains from other nonfermentative gram-negative bacilli.

It then becomes necessary to evaluate the findings on the basis of the identification techniques that were employed by the investigator. Some of the problems that have been encountered are discussed in detail by Schroth et al. and Hoadley in this monograph.

The development of precise techniques has paved the way for a clear understanding of the whole ecological niche of *P. aeruginosa* in the environment, plants and man. The portion of the niche that it occupies as a plant pathogen is economically important to the farmer or the green grocer who may suffer damage to his produce. It is also important to the commercial greenhouse owner who may experience "epidemics" caused by this organism among his plants. Schroth makes an interesting comparison between commercial greenhouses and hospitals as environments with similar problems of contraction and dissemination of disease agents. Both provide a closed environment in which contaminated water plays an important role in the epidemics that can occur. It still cannot be determined with certainty whether this role is chiefly that of the vehicle which spreads *P. aeruginosa* to plants, animals, or man, or whether water is a normal habitat for the organism. However, it is clear that this bacterium thrives in moist environments and is abundant in surface waters in warmer climates. As pointed out by Hoadley, the waters in northern climates with large populations of *P. aeruginosa* are those that have been contaminated by waste from man or domestic animals. In warm climates, there is evidence that this bacterium can proliferate in waters with high organic content in the absence of human or animal waste contamination. Its presence in soil may explain the increase in numbers in streams following rains and also provides a source of entry into greenhouses.

An interesting corollary occurs in the behavior of *P. aeruginosa* in its role as a disease-producing agent in plants and in humans. Under certain conditions of temperature and humidity, this bacterium colonizes plants without causing an apparent injury to the host. When these conditions are altered, it becomes an "opportunistic" pathogen that is then capable of producing disease. *P. aeruginosa* can also colonize man; then if host defenses become altered, it again assumes the role of an "opportunistic" pathogen and infection ensues.

Persons who receive organ transplant therapy as well as those with severe underlying diseases, such as cystic fibrosis, hematological malignancies, and those with severe trauma, extensive burns, etc., are at greater risk of infection with *P. aeruginosa*. It is the advent of new therapies that prolong the life of such patients but that compromise the defense systems against infection by use of corticosteroids, immunosuppressive agents, and cancer chemotherapeutic agents that render the host more susceptible to this bacterium. *P. aeruginosa* is often the leading cause of infectious death in patients with acute nonlymphocytic leukemia who are immunosuppressed and whose white blood cell count has been drastically lowered by chemotherapy. This organism has also long been a grim opponent to the survival of persons who have been hospitalized with extensive burns. The burned surfaces with their fluid accumulation provide an ideal medium for the growth of microorganisms, and the ubiquitous *P. aeruginosa* is, all too frequently, the bacterium that grows there in great abundance. Once a burn patient becomes colonized with *P. aeruginosa*, it is more difficult to prevent spread of the organism from patient to patient.

It is a truism that patients with compromised host defenses usually become infected with their own endogenous flora. At least two questions are raised by this statement. First, why *P. aeruginosa?* In other words, why is *P. aeruginosa*, which is not the most abundant organism in the host's flora, the one that is the most successful "opportunist?" Many pieces of the answer to this puzzle are presently under investigation, but the picture is not as yet complete. Second, what is the source of the endogenous flora that eventually infects the compromised host? Various investigators have placed the fecal carriage rate of *P. aeruginosa* in normal adults as ranging from about 3 to 19%. This rate rises rapidly upon hospitalization, and the likelihood of acquisition of an organism by each individual increases as the length of his hospital stay increases. Up to 47% of the microbiologically documented infections in patients with acute blood dyscrasias are caused by microorganisms acquired from the hospital environment. Such acquisition by patients during their hospital stay largely depends on their exposure to the organism; therefore, prevention of such exposure is a necessity.

Kominos and his co-workers demonstrated that it is possible to sharply reduce the acquisition of, and subsequent infection by, *P. aeruginosa* in hospitalized burn patients if proper preventive measures are instituted. The hospital kitchen must not be overlooked as a portal for bacterial exposure as vegetables contaminated with *P. aeruginosa* may arrive almost daily in this area. Fresh uncooked vegetables, a most desirable part of the diet for normal individuals, cannot safely be consumed by patients who are at high risk of infection by *P. aeruginosa.*

As described by Holder "a moist environment is the most common denominator of exogenous sources of *P. aeruginosa* in hospitals." From the nebulizers and humidifiers used in patient treatment, to the basins, sinks, and mops used for cleaning, these sources abound in hospitals. Virtually, any moist area in the hospital that is not kept decontaminated provides an area in which *P. aeruginosa* can survive or multiply and serves as a vehicle for patient exposure.

The question remains to be answered, how can it be that an organism such as *P. aeruginosa,* which colonizes only a small proportion of normal individuals and which requires the ingestion of large numbers to recover the organism from the feces, can so readily colonize certain hospitalized patients? Much of the information that we have on this subject is speculative and has been largely derived from the data developed on members of the *Enterobacteriaceae.* It has been established that suppression of normal enteric flora by antibiotics favors the growth of *P. aeruginosa* unless a specific anti-*Pseudomonas* agent is given; therefore, enteric flora must in some way restrict the growth of this bacterium, although the mode of suppressive action is not entirely clear. Levison's studies in mice provide a strong indication of one mechanism by which such suppression can take place and indicate a number of areas that are now only speculative but need delineation.

There is no explanation at this point for the tendency of specific serotypes to be predominant in a particular cancer group regardless of their prevalence in the total cancer patient population. As suggested by Moody, the intrinsic nature of specific serotypes also can influence the behavior of the microorganism in the host, in that one serotype could have a higher pathogenic potential than others. One of the serotypes she discusses appeared to have the characteristics of a "hospital strain."

Considerable research is presently underway to investigate properties of *P. aeruginosa* that determine its pathogenicity, but these studies are not included in this monograph. Nor is any attempt made to describe the newer developments in effective antibiotic therapy against this organism.

In concluding this introduction, it should be emphasized that a clear understanding of the cycles that this organism undergoes in the various environments in which it is found is an equally valid approach to the control of *P. aeruginosa*. As these cycles take place in such diverse environments as soil, plants, and water, a variety of disciplines must be brought together to effectuate control. Our knowledge of its ecology in soil and in surface waters has not yet been clearly defined and is still limited. Comprehension of the behavior of this bacterium in its varied niches must be developed before we understand the possible importance of these ecological sources in the transmission of *P. aeruginosa* to the hospitalized patient.

Pseudomonas aeruginosa: Ecological Aspects and Patient Colonization, edited by Viola Mae Young. Raven Press, New York © 1977.

Epidemiology of *Pseudomonas Aeruginosa* in Agricultural Areas

*Milton N. Schroth, *John J. Cho, *Sylvia K. Green, and **Spyros D. Kominos

*Department of Plant Pathology, University of California, Berkeley, California 94720; and** Microbiology Section, Mercy Hospital, Pittsburgh, Pennsylvania 15219

Most epidemiological studies of *Pseudomonas aeruginosa* have concerned the possible sources and mechanisms of transmission to patients in a hospital environment. These include solutions and creams, water faucets, incubators, milk formulas, sink drains, personnel, and inhalation and resuscitation equipment (4,6,12,17,25,28,52,64,66,81). These sources, however, probably represent transitory habitats rather than permanent or natural ones, and contamination is most likely from other origins. Following this line of thinking, we examined the possibility that soil and plants serve as the natural and permanent reservoirs for the bacterium. This seemed probable since it was described as a pathogen of lettuce (26,62), sugar cane (21), and tobacco (15,26). Unfortunately, this work is clouded because techniques were not available at the time of the studies to enable the investigators to differentiate between *P. aeruginosa* and other pseudomonads, such as *P. marginalis,* which are

1

plant pathogens. There is no doubt, however, of the validity of the *P. aeruginosa* strains that were described as pyocyanin positive (26).

Further evidence indicating that plants serve as a reservoir for *P. aeruginosa* and as an agent for dissemination emanates from the work of Shooter et al. (68,69), who found *P. aeruginosa* in hospital foods, and Kominos et al. (44), who isolated strains from vegetables that were indistinguishable from clinical strains on the basis of pyocin typing. These findings further suggest that *P. aeruginosa* is a common colonizer of vegetables and plants and may persist without causing symptoms. This is consistent with the findings of Samish and Etinger-Tulczynska (67) and others (3,48,73), who reported that some bacteria are normal inhabitants of plants and occur there without causing pathological conditions.

The concept that organisms such as *P. aeruginosa* might have the capacity to establish themselves in both plant and animal tissues has not been readily accepted because of the great difference in the structure, composition, and other intrinsic characteristics of the two forms of life (26). Nevertheless, some early work (5) suggested that *Sporotrichum schenkii,* which causes a human disease, also caused a rot of carnations and rosebuds. Ciferri and Baldacci (14) further claimed that 17 of 22 human pathogenic fungi and 2 of 23 human pathogenic bacteria infected tomato fruits. Starr and Chatterjee (75) also reported that various bacterial human pathogens caused injury when inoculated into plants. These reports, however, should be viewed from the perspective that plants, as well as mice or guinea pigs, will often produce a strong localized reaction when inoculated with large dosages of a foreign organism. The symptoms elicited from such inoculations may result from the artificiality of the experimentation and should not necessarily be considered indicative of the capacity of an organism to cause disease or colonize a host.

Unusual responses to inoculations frequently occur in plants when they are grown under unfavorable or abnormal environmental conditions since resistance mechanisms to invasion by microorganisms may be impaired. Differentiation can be made between the pathogen that produces disease by its ability to invade or penetrate the defenses of the normal host and the pathogen that is "opportunistic" and only attacks when host defenses are weakened. To test the capability of human pathogens to colonize plants or cause disease, the host should be grown under favorable environmental conditions before and after inoculation, followed by careful examination of the ability of an organism to invade, colonize tissue, or elicit a disease reaction, as differentiated from a mass reaction, at the site of inoculation.

When developing control strategies for a pathogen of animals or plants, it is important to have a good understanding of the biology and ecology of the organism in its various habitats, especially in those that are natural and permanent. In a field related to medical microbiology, plant pathology, the study of plant pathogens in their natural habitats has provided useful information for controlling pathogens in other environments. The natural "home" of the pathogen is also where one finds the greatest expression of the variability of a species, thus providing an indication of the strains that may eventually be disseminated to other localities such as greenhouses. Commercial greenhouses have points in common with hospitals, as they are also confronted with problems of preventing the contraction of disease and dissemination of the causal agent. Thus, to maintain a disease-free greenhouse, it is important to have an understanding of the epidemiology of pathogens: how they gain ingress into the greenhouse and how they are disseminated. After ingress, there are problems of dealing with drug resistance, determining mechanisms of transmission, and initiating control practice through the administration of antibiotics and chemicals.

This report summarizes the findings of our previous work on the epidemiology of *P. aeruginosa* in agricultural areas (13,35) and reviews some of the principal procedures for its isolation and identification. Our objectives were to examine the spectrum of strains occurring in nature, their distribution, their relationship to clinical strains, and the environmental conditions that favored their colonization of plants.

PROCEDURES FOR RECOVERY OF *P. AERUGINOSA* FROM SOIL AND PLANTS

Isolation

Various techniques for isolating *P. aeruginosa* have been developed and evolved with successive modifications by investigators (7,9,10,36,37,46,50,51, 58,70,72,78). The success and usefulness of these techniques depend, in part, on the nature of the sampling material. The selective isolation of *P. aeruginosa* is more difficult when the sampling material is soil, plant refuse, or plants because of the occurrence of a great variety of fluorescent pseudomonads with diverse nutritional characteristics in contrast to those found in specialized environments such as faucets or resuscitators. Accordingly, isolation techniques that are based on media with low selectivity do not enable a rapid differentiation of *P. aeruginosa* from other bacteria that may grow on the media. In order to increase such selectivity, various physical factors, and chemicals to which the organism is tolerant, have been used (7,10,37,42,46,51,70,78).

Our general procedure for isolating *P. aeruginosa* from soil and plants (35) was to place the sample in an enrichment medium consisting of acetamide and salts (70) and then to make a tenfold dilution series. After 48 hr incubation at 42°C, 0.1 ml of each suspension was placed on King's Medium B (42) supplemented with 0.03% cetrimide (KBC) (10) and followed by incubation at 42°C. Although a few pseudomonads and other bacteria may grow under these conditions, the colonies that fluoresce under UV were identified, almost without exception, as *P. aeruginosa*. The key factors in the selectivity of King's Medium B are the addition of KBC and incubation at 42°C. These two factors might also be useful supplements to the MacConkey agar (7), recently recommended for detection of *P. aeruginosa*.

Identification

When reviewing investigations on the epidemiology of bacterial species, especially those that are soil borne with many closely related species, the likelihood for error in strain and species identification increases relative to the age of the report. Thus, as previously stated, much of the early work concerning the capacity of *P. aeruginosa* to cause diseases of plants and insects (76) is moot because of the absence of definitive characteristics for differentiation among fluorescent pseudomonads; some early workers had particular difficulty in identifying *P. aeruginosa* when the strains were nonpigmented or produced fluorescein but not pyocyanin.

Various studies (1,11,29,31,32,63,74,77,80) have identified a number of useful diagnostic tests for differentiating *P. aeruginosa* from other pseudomonads. We found the following combination of tests particularly useful when identifying strains isolated from soil and plant materials: growth and fluorescein production at 42°C in acetamide and on KBC with or without pyocyanin production, growth on geraniol (74), positive oxidase test (31,32), and monotrichous flagellation (31,32). Additional tests employed were slime production in 2-ketogluconate (36), denitrification (74), and the inability to produce acids from disaccharides (32). The first two of these tests, however, have been reported to give variable results.

In our investigations, we generally ignored nonpigmented strains growing on KBC, because the few nonpigmented strains that grew on KBC in preliminary studies proved not to be *P. aeruginosa*. Many of these strains, however, produced fluorescein when grown at temperatures below 42° C.

Pyocin Typing

Definitive methods for the intraspecific identification of *P. aeruginosa* have evolved to the point where considerable confidence may be placed on the identity of strains. Pyocin typing as an accurate method for strain identification has greatly improved from the pioneer work of Jacob (40) and Holloway (39) with successive modifications and innovations (18,19,20,24,25,27,33, 34,53,55,57,59,79,82,83). Although both pyocin production (27,33,82) and pyocin sensitivity (27,61) may be used for typing, Bobo et al. (6) found the latter technique to be less stable, since strains that dissociated exhibited different sensitivity patterns.

Pyocin production appears to provide stable epidemiological markers when properly controlled, as erratic results among and within laboratories are likely to result from the absence of standardized procedures (34,57). For example, Govan and Gillies (34) observed that aberrant results occurred unless incubation of the strains to be typed was done with fairly strict limits on the temperature and the period of incubation. Merrikin and Terry (57) further recommended that the indicator inoculum be grown under a rigid schedule when typing strains and that indicator strains be lyophilized to prevent dissociations and mutations. Furthermore, the Darrell and Wahba method of pyocin typing (19) established such large major types that there was not sufficient specificity for adequate epidemiological tracking of the various strains. Zabransky and Day (82) used an additional set of indicator strains that enabled them to further differentiate the major types into subtypes. This modification has been used successfully in our studies (13,35) as well as in others (43,44).

Combined serological pyocin typing appears to offer the most reliable, sensitive, and precise ordering of *P. aeruginosa* strains. Although serological and pyocin typings have resulted in the derivation of similar conclusions in epidemiological studies when used properly (6), there are times when greater definition may be necessary. Accordingly, Csiszár and Lányi (18) reported that 543 strains

of *P. aeruginosa* from diverse sources could be subdivided according to O and H antigens into 53 serotypes
and 16 other, not fully defined, serological units using the
Lányi method (47). These serological units were subsequently subdivided into 165 combined seropyocin
types with a majority of serotypes containing two or
more different pyocin types. There also was an association between O antigen groups and pyocin types.

In our studies, strain identification of *P. aeruginosa*
was made on the basis of pyocin production for purposes of utility, although it would have been instructive
to have combined it with serotyping. Typing was based
on the inhibition patterns developed by Darrell and
Wahba (19) as modified by Zabransky and Day (82).

OCCURRENCE OF *P. AERUGINOSA* IN PLANTS, SOIL, AND WATER

Ornamental Plants

The frequency of recovery of *P. aeruginosa* from soil
supports the premise that it is a natural habitat of the
bacterium. Our investigations revealed that agricultural
soils and potted ornamental plants frequently harbored
P. aeruginosa (13,35). A summary of data to date is presented in Table 1. *P. aeruginosa* was readily isolated
from 41 of the 49 samples of potting soil, from 7 of 8
ornamental plants tested, as well as from some of the
steamed potting soils that had not been used for planting.
The soil generally contained 100 to 1,000 colony-forming
units (CFU) per gram of soil (13). Plant parts of six ornamental plants were tested for *P. aeruginosa*. Of the 199

plant parts of chrysanthemums tested, 50% harbored populations of *P. aeruginosa* at approximately 2 to 5 CFU per leaf. However, the incidence of infestation was related to the environmental conditions of plant culture. The percentage of plant parts with the bacterium was markedly less when they were maintained in retail houses, as the relative humidity (RH) was approximately 10 to 20% in contrast to the RH of 90 to 100% found in nursery propagation houses. The incidence of *P. aeruginosa* on other ornamental plants was much less than on chrysanthemums, and many were apparently free of the bacterium.

TABLE 1. *Summary of the incidence of* P. aeruginosa
in soil and plant material

| | No. samples positive/total | |
Source	Soil	Plant parts[a]
Ornamental plants		
African violet[b]	15/15	1/20
Aster beds	0/4	—
Azalea[b]	2/2	0/30
Begonia beds	0/9	—
Carnation beds	0/5	—
Chrysanthemum[b]	17/21	99/199
Dieffenbachia[b]	1/1	—
Fern[b]	—	0/10
Hydrangea[b]	2/2	0/40
Petunia[b]	4/5	3/15
Potting soil[c]	4/6	—
Rhododendron[b]	0/3	—
Rose bed	1/1	—
Tigredia beds	0/4	—

continued

TABLE 1—*continued*

Source	No. samples positive/total	
	Soil	Plant parts[a]
Crop plants		
Artichoke	0/6	—
Broccoli	0/1	—
Cabbage	0/1	—
Cauliflower	0/3	0/45
Celery	1/11	1/175
Corn	1/2	4/4
Cotton	1/1	—
Garlic	0/1	—
Lettuce	0/12	0/200
Onion	0/2	—
Potato	0/1	—
Spinach	0/1	0/50
Sugar beets	1/5	—
Tomato	11/24	0/475
Tomato leaves	—	1/875
Virgin soil[d]	1/2	—

[a] The vegetable samples were the edible portions such as the tomato fruit and the stalk of celery with the exception of corn where *P. aeruginosa* was isolated from the stalks.

[b] Plants were grown in pots rather than in beds or agricultural fields.

[c] Samples were from steamed potting soil mixtures prepared for planting.

[d] Soil was from an uncultivated area never used for agricultural purposes.

Crop Plants and Populations of *P. aeruginosa* in Soil

In contrast to the relatively high incidence of *P. aeruginosa* in ornamental plants and potted soil, much less was found in farm soils and crop plants (Tables 1 and 2). It was recovered from 15 to 71 farm soil samples. However, only 2 of 945 samples of edible plant parts, 1 of 575 tomato leaves, and 4 of 4 corn stalks sampled at the soil line. In contrast to the generally accepted premise that *P. aeruginosa* is associated with the activities of man, one of two soil samples from virgin soil (an uncultivated area never used for agricultural purposes) also yielded this organism.

Water

California farmlands are commonly irrigated with well water free of *P. aeruginosa,* at least at the well source (35). Such well water taken from several outlets as well as additional sources of water such as tap water and Colorado river water, were examined for the presence of *P. aeruginosa* by filtering 300 to 800 ml of water through a 0.22 μm Millipore filter, then culturing the filter in acetamide broth. The broth was then plated on KBC as previously described. Well water, which was free of *P. aeruginosa* when it was sampled at the origin, was frequently contaminated with *P. aeruginosa* after being drawn through hoses, fountains, and faucets (Table 3).

TABLE 2. Populations of P. aeruginosa in soil from different agricultural sources[a]

Source[b]	No. of soil samples	No. of samples with P. aeruginosa (population/g of soil)					
		10^0–10^1	10^1–10^2	10^2–10^3	10^3–10^4	10^4–10^5	10^5–10^6
Ornamental plants							
African violet	15			15			
Azalea	2			2			
Chrysanthemum	17			10	2	4	1
Hydrangea	2			2			
Petunia	4			4			
Potting soil	3			2	1		
Farmlands							
Celery	1	1					
Corn	1		1				
Cotton	1	1					
Tomato	10	2	4				

[a]Data represent soil samples listed in Table 1 where quantitative analyses of populations were made.

[b]The soils were from the pots of ornamental plants grown in different nurseries and farmlands of designated plants; potting soil refers to steam pasteurized soil prepared for planting.

Seven of 23 such sources of water contained *P. aeruginosa*. The bacterium was also detected in ditch water that emanated from a well that was devoid of *P. aeruginosa*. Water outlets in agricultural areas, faucets, fountains, etc., presumably become contaminated with *P. aeruginosa* because they come into contact with dust, soil, and other materials that carry the bacterium.

Pyocin Types

The pyocin types of *P. aeruginosa* that were isolated from plant, soil, and water samples are presented in Table 4. Assuming that plants and soil are natural reservoirs for *P. aeruginosa,* the high number of nontypable strains was not an unexpected finding, as isolations from these sources would provide a more representative sample of the diversity of the species in contrast to isolations

TABLE 3. *Incidence of* P. aeruginosa *in water collected from various agricultural areas*

Source	Location	No. sampled	No. positive
Nursery	Drinking fountains[a]	2	1
Nursery	Faucets[a]	7	3
Nursery	Hoses[a]	6	1
Nursery	Hose[b]	1	0
Nursery	Irrigation pipe[c]	1	1
Sugar beet field	Ditch[a]	1	1
Sugar beet field	Pump[a]	5	0
Total		23	7

[a] Well water.
[b] Colorado River water.
[c] Well water with inorganic fertilizer.

TABLE 4. Summary of pyocin types of P. aeruginosa isolates from water, soil, and plant material

Source	No. isolates typed	B-6	B-7	D-2	D-5	D-9	E-6	F-2	F-4	F-6	I-1	K	O	R-1	S	T	X-1	X-10	VT[a]	NT[b]
African violet foliage	6																		1	5
African violet soil	20										2									18
Azalea soil	3																			3
Chrysanthemum foliage	76	2	20	3				6	4	10	2	4	1		2				4	18
Chrysanthemum soil	44			1															6	37
Celery soil	1	1																		
Celery stalk	1															1				
Corn soil	2	1				1														
Cotton soil	1																			1
Hydrangea soil	9																			9
Petunia foliage	3																			3
Steam-treated soil	1												1							
Sugar beet soil	1																		1	
Tomato leaf	1		1																	
Tomato soil	28		7	10	1									1			3	1		5
Ditch water	1																1			
Fountain water	1					1														
Irrigation water	1																		1	
Total	200	4	28	14	1	1	1	6	4	10	4	4	2	1	2	1	4	1	13	99

[a] VT, variable type: unstable typing pattern.
[b] NT, nontypable: no inhibition of indicator strains.

14

from more specialized environments. Many of the isolates from the foliage of chrysanthemums, petunias, and
African violets, as well as the soil of various plants, were
nontypable. The exception was a tomato field where
most of the isolates were typable. The typing also revealed the presence of the pyocin types B-7, D-2, F-2,
and F-6, which are also frequently isolated from clinical
specimens (43,44). Some of the isolates, furthermore,
were resistant to carbenicillin (35).

Colonization of Plants by *P. aeruginosa*

Plants are commonly colonized with *P. aeruginosa,*
although they may represent a somewhat transitory environment for the bacterium. The population of the bacterium in plants declines rapidly when they are grown
under conditions of low moisture. Plants most likely are
colonized only under special environmental conditions.
As demonstrated in the experiments of Green et al. (35),
P. aeruginosa could multiply when inoculated into lettuce and bean plants grown at 80 to 95% relative humidity and 27°C, but approached a steady state at that temperature when the RH was reduced to 55 to 75%. At the
latter condition, there was no evidence of disease or injury to the inoculated leaves. The scarcity of *P.
aeruginosa* in agricultural plants from semiarid areas in
California, and the similarly low incidence of recovery of
this organism from retail outlets, in contrast to the numbers found in propagation houses with high humidity,
further demonstrates the necessity of high levels of
humidity for colonization and survival of *P. aeruginosa*
in plant tissues.

Pathogenicity of *P. aeruginosa* in Plants

The plant pathogenicity of various strains of *P. aeruginosa* that had been isolated from different sources, such as clinical specimens, plants, soil, and water, was tested by inoculating vegetables with 24 hr old cultures that had been suspended in sterile distilled water to a concentration of approximately 10^8 cells/ml, as previously described (35). The vegetables used were lettuce slices (*Lactuca sativa* L. "Great Lakes"), celery stalks (*Apium graveolens* L. var. Dulce), potato tuber slices (*Solanum tuberosum* L. "Whiterose"), tomato (*Lycopersicon esculentum* L. Mill), cucumber (*Cucumis sativus* L.), rutabaga (*Brassica campestris* L.), and carrot (*Daucus carrota* L. var. *sativa*). Inoculated vegetables were incubated at 28°C at approximately 100% RH, observed daily, and symptoms recorded at approximately 72 hr after inoculation. Although preliminary studies indicated that inocula concentrations of $> 10^3$ cells/ml incited disease, greater dosages were used in these tests because of the uniformity of results and the rapidity with which symptoms developed.

There was considerable variation in the capacity of *P. aeruginosa* to incite rot of the vegetables (Table 5 and Fig. 1). This variability was not related to the source of the strains or the pyocin type, as the rot incited by clinical isolates was indistinguishable from that caused by agricultural isolates. The amount of rot varied among strains from both sources with some inciting rot and others little to none. Some isolates appeared to cause localized areas of water soaking that became discolored from pigment produced by the bacterium (Fig. 2); these symptoms were usually not accompanied by rot. Al-

TABLE 5. Capacity of P. aeruginosa to incite rot of vegetable materials[a]

Source and isolate no.	Pyocin type	Bean	Brussel sprout	Carrot	Celery	Cucumber	Lettuce	Potato	Rutabaga	Tomato
Clinical										
PA-3	D-2	1	1	1	2	4	3	3	1	2
PA-4	B-7	4	1	0	0	3	4	4	1	1
PA-5	B-3	3	2	1	1	4	3	3	1	3
PA-6	E-7	3	1	1	1	2	2	2	1	3
PA-7	J-6	3	1	1	1	3	3	3	1	3
PA-10	B-7	2	1	1	1	2	4	3	2	4
PA-11	F-6	0	1	0	1	0	3	0	1	0
PA-12	F-6	1	1	2	1	3	1	1	1	3
PA-13	B-4	3	1	2	1	4	4	4	1	4
PA-14	E-6	2	1	3	2	3	4	4	2	3
PA-37	K	3	1	3	2	3	4	3	1	4
PA-38	D-2	3	1	3	2	3	3	3	1	4
PA-39	F-2	4	1	2	2	3	2	2	1	4
PA-40	F-2	2	1	3	1	3	3	2	1	3
PA-41	VT	2	3	3	2	3	3	3	1	3
PA-42	D-2	3	1	3	2	3	3	2	1	3
PA-43	E-7	3	2	2	2	3	3	3	1	3
PA-44	VT	3	1	2	1	2	3	2	1	4
PA-45	A-3	3	1	3	1	3	3	3	1	3
PA-46	D-2	2	1	1	2	3	3	0	1	3
PA-47	0-2	2	1	2	1	3	3	3	1	3
Plant										
PA-16	NT	2	2	1	1	3	2	4	1	3
PA-17	NT	4	1	1	2	4	3	4	1	3

continued

17

TABLE 5—continued

Source and isolate no.	Pyocin type	Bean	Brussel sprout	Carrot	Celery	Cucumber	Lettuce	Potato	Rutabaga	Tomato
PA-18	NT	3	1	1	1	3	3	3	1	2
PA-19	NT	3	2	1	1	3	3	4	1	3
PA-20	NT	1	1	0	1	1	3	2	1	3
PA-21	NT	2	1	1	1	1	2	0	1	2
PA-22	NT	2	1	0	1	—	2	0	1	2
PA-23	B-7	2	2	2	1	3	3	2	1	2
PA-24	B-7	3	2	2	1	3	3	2	1	3
PA-25	B-7	3	2	2	2	3	3	2	1	3
PA-26	F-6	3	1	3	1	3	4	3	1	3
PA-27	F-2	3	3	3	2	4	4	4	1	4
PA-28	F-6	4	1	2	2	3	4	3	1	3
PA-29	F-2	4	2	3	2	4	3	3	1	4
PA-30	F-2	4	1	2	2	4	4	3	1	4
PA-31	F-2	4	1	3	2	4	4	3	1	4
PA-32	F-2	2	1	3	2	3	3	3	1	3
PA-33	F-2	4	2	2	2	4	4	3	2	4
PA-50	F-6	2	2	1	2	3	3	3	1	3
PA-51	VT	2	2	3	1	4	2	3	1	2
PA-52	B-7	3	3	1	1	4	3	3	1	3
PA-53	B-7	3	1	1	1	3	2	3	1	3
PA-54	F-4	3	1	2	2	4	4	3	2	4
PA-55	0	1	1	1	0	3	2	2	1	3
PA-56	F-4	3	1	2	2	3	4	3	2	2
PA-58	I	3	1	2	2	3	4	3	1	4

Isolate	Source									
PA-59	K	2	1	1	1	1	2	2	1	3
PA-61	F-2	2	2	2	3	3	4	3	1	3
PA-62	D-2	3	1	2	2	4	4	3	1	4
PA-63	D-2	2	2	2	3	3	3	3	1	3
PA-64	D-2	2	1	2	1	3	4	2	1	3
PA-65	D-2	2	2	2	2	3	3	3	2	3
PA-66	D-2	3	2	2	2	3	3	2	1	3
Water										
W1	E-6	3	1	2	2	3	2	2	1	3
W3a	K	2	1	2	2	3	3	3	1	2
W3b	K	2	1	2	2	4	3	2	1	2
W4	VT	2	2	2	2	3	3	3	1	3
W5a	VT	2	1	2	2	3	2	2	1	3
W5b	VT	3	1	2	2	4	4	4	2	3
W5-17a	I-1	2	2	3	3	3	2	3	2	3
W18-18	X-1	2	2	2	2	3	2	3	1	2
Soil										
S5	K	3	1	2	2	3	2	2	1	3
S34-133	V-10	2	1	1	1	3	3	3	1	2
SB34-187	V-10	2	1	3	3	3	2	3	1	2
S5-17b	I-1	2	2	2	2	3	2	2	1	3
PA-35	VT	1	1	0	2	1	0	0	1	0
PA-57	F-6	3	1	3	3	3	4	4	1	3
PA-60	NT	1	1	1	1	1	2	1	1	1

[a]Pathogenicity tests were conducted at approximately 100% RH at 28°C. 0, no symptoms; 1, localized water soaking and discoloration of tissue around site of inoculation but no rotting of tissue; 2, moderate rot; 3, severe rot with much of the tissue softened; 4, complete rot of tissues.

19

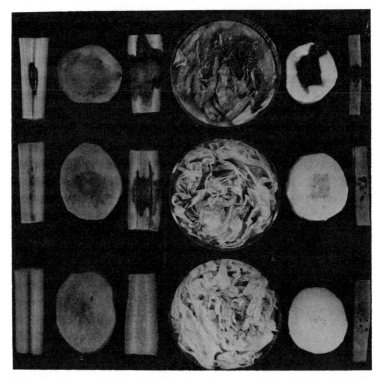

FIG. 1. Slices (left to right) of celery, potato, carrot, lettuce, rutabaga, and bean inoculated with *P. aeruginosa,* clinical strains PA-14 **(top row)**, PA-12 **(middle),** and control **(bottom row),** showing varying capacity to rot vegetables. Vegetable slices were incubated for 72 hr at 28°C.

though there were some indications of host specificity among the strains, a strain which exhibited virulence to one vegetable generally was just as virulent to others.

The results of these pathogenicity tests differed slightly from a previous study (35), primarily because of the lower temperature used for incubation. However,

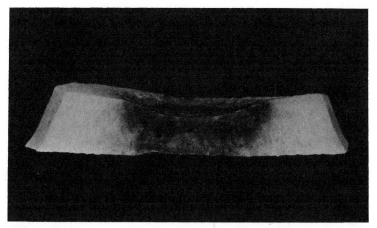

FIG. 2. Slice of rutabaga inoculated with *P. aeruginosa,* clinical strain PA-14, showing a depression at the site of inoculation and the diffusion of pyocyanin produced by the bacterium throughout the tissues.

this applied only to scoring the degrees of virulence and did not change the general pattern of response among strains from different sources. That strains from clinical specimens and agricultural materials both incited rot is strongly indicative of the similarity among the strains. Live plant materials represent a complex medium in which relatively few microorganisms can colonize or infect because of host-defense mechanisms. When an invasion occurs, there are also specific host responses that depend on the nature of the pathogen and the status of the host-defense mechanisms. Thus, the capability of *P. aeruginosa* strains from different sources to cause similar symptoms on the same host is strong evidence that the strains are either identical or closely related.

P. aeruginosa is not a typical plant pathogen since it

does not ordinarily cause macroscopic damage to plants, unless they are subjected to conditions of moderate to high temperature and high moisture. Furthermore, it has been reported that *P. aeruginosa* does not produce pectic enzymes (16,65) normally associated with pathogens that cause rot. In our tests using pectate gels (38), we also could not detect the presence of pectic enzymes, regardless of pH or incubation temperature. When investigating rotted vegetables that had been inoculated with *P. aeruginosa*, we consistently recovered soft-rotting bacteria such as *P. marginalis* and *Erwinia carotovora*. This suggests that *P. aeruginosa* may well cause rot through a synergistic action with other microflora that colonize vegetables.

DISCUSSION

Our studies and others (2,8,22,23,30,44,45,49, 54,56,60,71) on *Klebsiella, Enterobacter,* and the plant pathogen *P. cepacia* suggest that a number of human pathogens may survive and persist in a variety of environments. This points to the importance of extending studies on the etiology of nosocomial diseases from hospital environments to agricultural areas or other locations that may serve as natural reservoirs. The role of plants, vegetables, and other agents in disseminating and transmitting *P. aeruginosa* and other bacteria should be clearly researched as to its importance in contributing to nosocomial diseases. Kominos et al. (44) showed that fresh vegetables commonly carried strains of *P. aeruginosa* and considered them to be an important agent in contributing to the dissemination of the pathogen.

Although nurseries attempt to keep greenhouses free

from pathogens, the opportunity for *P. aeruginosa* to colonize ornamental plants has its origin in several greenhouse practices. For example, our investigations indicated that steamed and autoclaved soils used for pottings apparently were colonized by *P. aeruginosa* before planting, since no measures were taken to prevent contamination. In addition, *P. aeruginosa* was found in the water from hoses and faucets and in the combined water-fertilization solution used to irrigate plants. Lastly, cuttings brought into the propagation houses from the "mother block" that harbors the bacterium serve as a source of *P. aeruginosa* to contaminate other plants in the greenhouse.

Control

If necessary, controls could be devised to reduce the likelihood that plants and food materials brought into hospitals carry *P. aeruginosa*. Some of these controls could be applied in the growing areas. With present knowledge of the environmental conditions that favor multiplication and survival of *P. aeruginosa,* it should be possible for agriculturalists to reduce the chance of plants becoming infested with *P. aeruginosa* without having to make drastic and costly alterations of cultural procedures. Plants grown for consumption are less likely to be colonized by *P. aeruginosa* when grown in arid areas or in disease-free greenhouses. The conditions during processing, storage, and transit are also important in safeguarding against contamination by *P. aeruginosa*. The exposure of plant material to sources known to carry *P. aeruginosa,* such as soil or insects, coupled with conditions of high moisture during storage, create an ideal environment for invasion and colonization of plant tissues. This and other agricultural practices should be examined in relation to the role of food and plant materials as sources for *P. aeruginosa* and other potential pathogens of humans.

REFERENCES

1. Azuma, Y., and Witter, L. D. (1964): Pyocyanin formation by some normally apyocyanogenic strains of *Pseudomonas aeruginosa*. *J. Bacteriol.*, 87:1254.
2. Ballard, R. W., Palleroni, N. J., Doudoroff, M., and Stanier, R. Y. (1968); Taxonomy of the aerobic pseudomonads: *Pseudomonas cepacia, P. marginata, P. alliicola,* and *P. caryophylli. J. Gen. Microbiol.*, 60:199−214.
3. Barnes, E. H. (1965): Bacteria on leaf surfaces and in intercellular leaf spaces. *Science,* 147:1151−1152.
4. Bassett, D. J. C. (1971): Causes and prevention of sepsis due to gram negative bacteria: Common source outbreaks. *Proc. Roy. Soc. Med.*, 64:979−985.
5. Benham, R. W., and Kester, B. (1932): Sporotrichosis, its transmission to plants and animals. *J. Infect. Dis.*, 50:437−458.
6. Bobo, R. A., Newton, E. J., Jones, L. F., Farmer, L. H., and Farmer, J. J., III. (1973): Nursery outbreak of *Pseudomonas aeruginosa:* Epidemiological conclusions from five different typing methods. *Appl. Microbiol.*, 25:414−420.
7. Brodsky, M. H. and Nixon, M. C. (1973): Rapid method for detection of *Pseudomonas aeruginosa* on MacConkey agar under ultraviolet light. *Appl. Microbiol.*, 26:219−220.
8. Brown, C., and Seidler, R. J. (1973): Potential pathogens in the environment: *Klebsiella pneumoniae,* a taxonomic and ecological enigma. *Appl. Microbiol.*, 25:900−904.
9. Brown, M. R. W., and Foster, J. H. S. (1970): A simple diagnostic milk medium for *Pseudomonas aeruginosa. J. Clin. Pathol.*, 23:172−177.
10. Brown, V. I., and Lowbury, E. J. L. (1965): Use of an improved cetrimide agar medium and other culture methods for *Pseudomonas aeruginosa. J. Clin. Pathol. (London),* 18:752−756.
11. Bühlmann, X., Vischer, W. A., and Bruhin, H. (1961): Identifica-

tion of apyocyanogenic strains of *Pseudomonas aeroginosa. J. Bacteriol.,* 82:787–788.

12. Cartwright, R. Y., and Hargrove, P. R. (1970): *Pseudomonas* in ventilators. *Lancet,* 1:40.

13. Cho, J. J., Schroth, M. N., Kominos, S. D., and Green, S. K. (1975): Ornamental plants as carriers of *Pseudomonas aeruginosa. Phytopathology,* 65:425-431.

14. Ciferri, R., and Baldacci, E. (1934): Intorno alla pathogenicitá di alcuni miceti dell' uomo per il frutto del pomodoro. *Boll. Soc. Biol. Sper.,* 9:200–202.

15. Clara, F. M. (1930): A new bacterial leaf disease of tobacco in the Philippines. *Phytopathology,* 20:691–706.

16. Coles, H. W. (1926): The digestion of pectin and methylated glucoses by various organisms. *Plant Physiol.,* 1:379–385.

17. Cooke, E. M., Shooter, R. A., O'Farrell, S. M., and Martin, D. R. (1970): Faecal carriage of *Pseudomonas aeruginosa* by newborne babies. *Lancet,* 2:1045–1046.

18. Csiszár, K. and Lányi, B. (1970): Pyocine typing of *Pseudomonas aeruginosa* : Association between antigenic structure and pyocine type. *Acta Microbiol. Acad. Sci. Hung.,* 17:361–370.

19. Darrell, J. H., and Wahba, A. H. (1964): Pyocine-typing of hospital strains of *Pseudomonas pyocyanae. J. Clin. Pathol. (Lond.),* 17:236–242.

20. Deighton, M. A., Tagg, J. R., and Mushin, R. (1971): Epidemiology of *Pseudomonas aeruginosa* infection in hospitals. 2. "Fingerprinting" of *P. aeruginosa* strains in a study of cross-infection in a children's hospital. *Med. J. Aust.,* 1:892–896.

21. Desai, S. V. (1935): Stinking rot of sugarcane. *Indian J. Agric. Sci.,* 5:387–392.

22. Duncan, D. W., and Razzel, W. E. (1972): *Klebsiella* biotypes among coliforms isolated from forest environments and farm produce. *Appl. Microbiol.,* 24:933–938.

23. Ederer, G. M., and Matsen, J. M. (1972): Colonization and infection with *Pseudomonas cepacia. J. Infect. Dis.,* 125:613–618.

24. Edmonds, P., Suskind, R. R., MacMillan, B. G., and Holder, I. A. (1972): Epidemiology of *Pseudomonas aeruginosa* in a burns hospital: Evaluation of serological, bacteriophage, and pyocin typing methods. *Appl. Microbiol.,* 24:213–218.

25. Edmonds, P., Suskind, R. R., MacMillan, B. G., and Holder, I. A. (1972): Epidemiology of *Pseudomonas aeruginosa* in a burns hospital: Surveillance by a combined typing system. *Appl. Microbiol.,* 24:219–225.

26. Elrod, R. P., and Braun, A. C. (1942): *Pseudomonas aeruginosa:* Its role as a plant pathogen. *J. Bacteriol.,* 44:633–644.
27. Farmer, J. J., III, and Herman, L. G. (1969): Epidemiological fingerprinting of *Pseudomonas aeruginosa* by the production of and sensitivity to pyocin and bacteriophage. *Appl. Microbiol.,* 18:760–765.
28. Fierer, J., Taylor, P. M., and Gezon, H. M. (1967): *Pseudomonas aeruginosa* epidemic traced to a delivery room resuscitator. *N. Engl. J. Med.,* 276:991–996.
29. Gaby, W. L., and Free, E. (1958): Differential diagnosis of *Pseudomonas*-like micro-organisms in the clinical laboratory. *J. Bacteriol.,* 76:442–444.
30. Geldreich, E. E., Kenner, B. A., and Kabler, P. W. (1964): Occurrence of coliforms, fecal coliforms and streptococci on vegetation and insects. *Appl. Microbiol.,* 12:63–69.
31. Gilardi, G. L. (1968): Diagnostic criteria for differentiation of pseudomonads pathogenic for man. *Appl. Microbiol.,* 16:1497–1502.
32. Gilardi, G. L. (1971): Characterization of *Pseudomonas* species isolated from clinical specimens. *Appl. Microbiol.,* 21:414–419.
33. Gillies, R. R., and Govan, J. R. W. (1966): Typing of *Pseudomonas pyocyanea* by pyocine production. *J. Pathol. Bacteriol.,* 91:339–345.
34. Govan, J. R. W., and Gillies, R. H. (1969): Further studies on the pyocine typing of *Pseudomonas pyocyanea. J. Med. Microbiol.,* 2:17–25.
35. Green, S. K., Schroth, M. N., Cho J. J., and Kominos, S. D. (1974): Agricultural plants and soil as a possible reservoir for *Pseudomonas aeruginosa. Appl. Microbiol.,* 28:987–991.
36. Haynes, W. C. (1951): *Pseudomonas aeruginosa*—its characterization and identification. *J. Gen. Microbiol.,* 5:939–950.
37. Hedberg, M. (1969): Acetamide agar medium selective for *Pseudomonas aeruginosa. Appl. Microbiol.,* 17:481.
38. Hildebrand, D. C. (1971): Pectate and pectin gels for differentiation of *Pseudomonas* sp. and other bacterial plant pathogens. *Phytopathology,* 61:1430–1436.
39. Holloway, B. W. (1960): Grouping *Pseudomonas aeruginosa* by lysogenicity and pyocinogenicity. *J. Pathol. Bacteriol.,* 80:448–450.
40. Jacob, F. (1954): Bisynthèse induit et mode d'action d'une pyocine antibiotique de *Pseudomonas pyocyanea. Ann. Inst. Pasteur,* 86:149–160.
41. Kawamoto, S. O., and Lorbeer, J. W. (1974): Infection of onion

leaves by *Pseudomonas cepacia.* *Phytopathology,* 64:1440–1446.

42. King, E. O., Ward, M. K., and Raney, D. E. (1954): Two simple media for the demonstration of pyocyanin and fluorescein. *J. Lab. Clin. Med.,* 44:301–307.

43. Kominos, S. D., Copeland, C. E., and Grosiak, B. (1972): Mode of transmission of *Pseudomonas aeruginosa* in a burn unit and an intensive care unit in a general hospital. *Appl. Microbiol.,* 23:309–312.

44. Kominos, S. D., Copeland, C. E., Grosiak, B., and Postic, B. (1972): Introduction of *Pseudomonas aeruginosa* into a hospital via vegetables. *Appl. Microbiol.,* 24:567–570.

45. Knowles, R., Neufeld, R., and Simpson, S. (1974): Acetylene reduction (nitrogen fixation) by pulp and paper mill effluents and by *Klebsiella* isolated from effluents and environmental situations. *Appl. Microbiol.,* 28:608–613.

46. Lambe, D. W., Jr., and Stewart, P. (1972): Evaluation of pseudosel agar as an aid in the identification of *Pseudomonas aeruginosa. Appl. Microbiol.,* 23:377–381.

47. Lányi, B. (1970): Serological properties of *Pseudomonas aeruginosa.* II. Type-specific thermolabile (flagellar) antigens. *Acta Microbiol. Acad. Sci. Hung.,* 17:35–48.

48. Leben, C. (1974): Survival of plant pathogenic bacteria. *Ohio Agr. Res. and Develop. Ctr., Wooster, Ohio* (Special Circular), 100:21 pp.

49. Line, M. A. and Loutit, M. W. (1971): Non-symbiotic nitrogen-fixing organisms from some New Zealand tussock-grassland soils. *J. Gen. Microbiol.,* 66:309–318.

50. Lowbury, E. J. L. (1951): Improved culture methods for the detection of *Pseudomonas pyocyanea. J. Clin. Pathol.,* 4:66–72.

51. Lowbury, E. J. L., and Collins, A. E. (1955): The use of a new cetrimide product in a selective medium for *Pseudomonas pyocyanea. J. Clin. Pathol.,* 8:47–48.

52. Lowbury, E. J. L., Thom, B. T., Lilly, H. A., Babb, J. R., and Whittall, K. (1970): Sources of infection with *Pseudomonas aeruginosa* in patients with tracheostomy. *J. Med. Microbiol.,* 3:39–56.

53. MacPherson, J. N., and Gillies, R. R. (1969): A note on bacteriocine typing techniques. *J. Med. Microbiol.,* 2:161–165.

54. Matsen, J. M., Spindler, J. A., and Blosser, R. O. (1974): Characterization of *Klebsiella* isolates from natural receiving waters and comparison with human isolates. *Appl. Microbiol.,* 28:672–678.

55. Matsumoto, H., Tazaki, T., and Kato, T. (1968): Serological and

pyocine types of *Pseudomonas aeruginosa* from various sources. *Jpn. J. Microbiol.*, 12:111−119.

56. McCoy, R. H., and Seidler, R. J. (1973): Potential pathogens in the environment: Isolatin, enumeration, and identification of seven genera of intestinal bacteria associated with small green pet turtles. *Appl. Microbiol.*, 25:534−538.

57. Merrikin, D. J., and Terry, C. S. (1972): Variability of pyocine type and pyocine sensitivity in some strains of *Pseudomonas aeruginosa*. *J. Appl. Bact.*, 35:667−672.

58. National Communicable Disease Center (1967): Laboratory methods in special bacteriology. Course ≋8390-C, NCDC, Atlanta, Ga.

59. Neussil, H. (1971): Die Bedeutung der Pyocin-Typisierung bei Kontrollen des Verlaufes von Harnweginfektionen mit *Pseudomonas aeruginosa*. *Arzneim. Forsch.*, 21:333−335.

60. Nunez, W. J., and Colmer, A. R. (1968): Differentiation of *Aerobacter-Klebsiella* isolated from sugarcane. *Appl. Microbiol.*, 16:1875−1878.

61. Osman, M. A. M. (1965): Pyocine typing of *Pseudomonas aeruginosa*. *J. Clin. Pathol.*, 18:200−202.

62. Paine, S. G., and Branfoot, J. M. (1924): Studies in bacteriosis. XI. A bacterial disease of lettuce. *Ann. Appl. Biol.*, 11:312−317.

63. Plase, M., Malcolm, J., Chernaik, R., and Dunlop, S. (1968): An approach to the problem of differentiating Pseudomonads in the clinical laboratory. *Am. J. Med. Technol.*, 34:35−40.

64. Phillips, I., and Spenser, G. (1965): *Pseudomonas aeruginosa:* Cross infection due to contaminated respirator apparatus. *Lancet*, 2:1325−1327.

65. Prunier, J. P., and Kaiser, ,P. (1964): Study on the pectinolytic activity in phytopathogenic and saprophytic bacteria of plants. I. Research on pectinolytic enzymes. *Ann. Epiphyt.*, 15:205−219.

66. Rees, T. A. (1970): Bacteria in suction machines. *Lancet*, 1:240.

67. Samish, Z., and Etinger-Tulczynska, R. (1963): Distribution of bacteria within the tissue of healthy tomatoes. *Appl. Microbiol.*, 11:7−10.

68. Shooter, R. A., Cooke, E. M., Faiers, M. C., Breaden, A. L., and O'Farrell, S. M. (1971): Isolation of *Escherichia coli, Pseudomonas aeruginosa,* and *Klebsiella* from food in hospitals, canteens, and schools. *Lancet*, 2:390−392.

69. Shooter, R. A., Gaya, H., Cooke, E. M., Kumar, P., Patel, N., Parker, M. T., Thom, B. T., and France, D. R. (1969): Food and medicaments as possible sources of hospital strains of *Pseudomonas aeruginosa*. *Lancet*, 1:1227−1229.

70. Smith, R. F., and Dayton, S. L. (1972): Use of acetamide broth in the isolation of *Pseudomonas aeroginosa* from rectal swabs. *Appl. Microbiol.*, 24:143–145.
71. Snell, J. J. S., Hill, L. R., Lapage, S. P., and Curtis, M. A. (1972): Identification of *Pseudomonas cepacia* Burkholder and its synonomy with *Pseudomonas kingii* Jonsson. *Int. J. Systemat. Bacteriol.*, 22:127–138.
72. Solari, A. A., Dato, A. A., Herrero, M. M., de Cremaschi, M. S. D., de Reid, M. I., Salgado, L. P., and Painceira, M. T. (1962): Use of a selective enrichment medium for the isolation of *Pseudomonas aeruginosa* from feces. *J. Bacteriol.*, 84:190.
73. Stanghellini, M. E. (1972): Bacterial seed-piece decay and blackleg of potato. *Prog. Agr. in Arizona*, 24:4, 5, 16.
74. Stanier, R. Y., Palleroni, N. J., and Duodoroff, M. (1966): The aerobic pseudomonads: A taxonomic study. *J. Gen. Microbiol.*, 43:159–271.
75. Starr, M. P., and Chatterjee, A. K. (1972): The genus Erwinia: Enterobacteria pathogenic to plants and animals. *Ann. Rev. Microbiol.*, 26:389–426.
76. Steinhaus, E. A. (1949): *Principles of Insect Pathology*, p. 308. McGraw-Hill Book Co., Inc., New York.
77. Sutter, V. (1968): Identification of *Pseudomonas* species isolated from hospital environments and human sources. *Appl. Microbiol.*, 16:1532–1538.
78. Thom, A. R., Stephens, M. E., Gillespie, W. A., and Alder, V. G. (1971): Nitrofurantoin media for the isolation of *Pseudomonas aeruginosa. J. Appl. Bacteriol.*, 34:611–614.
79. Wahba, A. H. (1965): Hospital and infection with *Pseudomonas pyocyanea:* An investigation by a combined pyocine and serological typing method. *Brit. Med. J.*, 1:86–89.
80. Wahba, A. H., and Darrell, J. H. (1965): The identification of atypical strains of *Pseudomonas aeruginosa. J. Gen. Microbiol.*, 38:329–342.
81. Whitby, J. L., and Rampling, A. (1972): *Pseudomonas aeruginosa* contamination in domestic and hospital environments. *Lancet*, 1:15–17.
82. Zabransky, R. J., and Day, F. E. (1969): Pyocine-typing of clinical strains of *Pseudomonas aeruginosa. Appl. Microbiol.*, 17:293–296.
83. Ziv, G., Mushin, R., and Tagg, J. R. (1971): Pyocine typing as an epidemiological marker in *Pseudomonas aeruginosa* mastitis in cattle. *J. Hyg.*, 69:171–177.

Pseudomonas aeruginosa: Ecological Aspects and Patient Colonization, edited by Viola Mae Young. Raven Press, New York © 1977.

Pseudomonas aeruginosa in Surface Waters

Alfred W. Hoadley

School of Civil Engineering, Georgia Institute of Technology, Atlanta, Georgia 30332

Pseudomonas aeruginosa is considered a ubiquitous bacterial species easily isolated from surface waters and soil and able to infect a variety of plants, as well as man and animals. That the species can be isolated from soil and surface waters has been amply demonstrated. On the other hand, the extent to which *P. aeruginosa* may be considered a normal inhabitant of these environments is not clear, and it probably can be regarded as part of the autochthonous flora of surface waters only under special conditions.

However, water may play a major role in the dissemination of *P. aeruginosa* in the environment, carrying the organisms to man, animals, and plants. The spread by irrigation water of other pseudomonads pathogenic to plants has been reported (28). Plants in turn may serve as vehicles for the transmission of *P. aeruginosa* to man (34,56,57,62).

Waterborne outbreaks of *P. aeruginosa* infections in animals are well documented. Among such outbreaks are waterborne bovine mastitis (7,10,25,41,48,50),

31

pneumonia in calves (49), and infections in mink (3,64), chinchillas (38), and rabbits (42). Mushin and Ziv (46) found a high incidence (80.1%) of pyocin type 1 *P. aeruginosa* associated with bovine mastitis on farms in Israel that reflected a predominance of the type in the environment, including water samples.

Infections in man also have been reported following contact with surface waters. Cothran and Hatlen (9) reported isolation of *P. aeruginosa* from swimming pool water and from the infected outer ears of swimmers at the pool. Favero et al. (15) later reported that, by phage typing, Hoff had established the identity of strains isolated from the pool water and from infected ears. Furthermore, in limited studies of infected outer ears of swimmers at pools in Florida (22), *P. aeruginosa* strains of identical immunotype and pyocin type were isolated from pool waters and infected outer ears of two swimmers. Identical strains of fluorescent pseudomonads capable of growth at 41°C but differing from *P. aeruginosa* were also isolated from pool waters and the infected and healthy auditory canals of two swimmers. *Pseudomonas aeruginosa* infections of wounds sustained in contaminated aquatic environments have been described; most recently, D. Taplin *(unpublished report)* reported on infections among survivors of a plane crash in the Everglades and in a 17-year-old girl severely injured in a boating accident.

Although contamination of moist environments in hospitals, and the subsequent growth of *P. aeruginosa,* would ordinarily appear to be traceable to fecal carriers or infected patients, *P. aeruginosa* may enter the hospital directly or indirectly by way of water supplies. Hunter and Ensign (29) attributed an epidemic of diarrhea in a newborn nursery to contamination of the milk supply. At one milk plant supplying the hospital, *P. aeruginosa* entered the pasteurized milk from a leaking water pipe wrapped with a rag which dripped into the cooling vats. In more recently reported episodes, water supplies have been shown to constitute reservoirs of *P. aeruginosa* and sources of contamination in hospital environments. *Pseudomonas aeruginosa* was isolated from the taps of eight washing sinks in an operating theater of one hospital with a cold water supply consisting of open roof tanks that were fouled by birds and contained two dead pigeons (63). Weber et al. (65) reported an epidemic of *P. aeruginosa* infections in a newborn nursery that was caused by a well-water supply contaminated by seepage of sewage and infiltration of contaminated stream water.

ENUMERATION OF *P. AERUGINOSA*

A variety of methods has been employed to demonstrate *P. aeruginosa* in surface and drinking waters and to estimate populations. Most probable numbers (MPNs) are used most commonly. Ringen and Drake (52) applied the MPN technique first, employing a modification of Burton's medium containing pyocyanin that was highly selective for *P. aeruginosa*. After 96 hr incubation at 37°C, cells were transferred from enrichment media to agar slants of the basal medium without pyocyanin for confirmation of pyocyanin production. Reitler and Seligmann (51) later inoculated drinking water samples into bile salt, lactose, peptone, and water incubated for 48 hr at 37°C. Following incubation, the broths were streaked onto "plain agar" plates that were observed for pyocyanin production after incubation for 24 hr at 37°C.

The latter procedure permitted simultaneous enumeration of *P. aeruginosa* and *Escherichia coli.* Recently, Clark and Vlassoff (8) employed enrichments in Mac-Conkey broth modified by the addition of 5 g Tryptone per liter to demonstrate simultaneously the presence or absence of *P. aeruginosa* and other indicator bacteria in drinking water samples. Enrichments in modified Mac-Conkey broth were incubated at 35°C for up to 5 days, after which cells were transferred to the liquid medium 10 of Drake (11), which was incubated at 35°C for 2 to 4 days. Cells from tubes exhibiting fluorescence were streaked on MacConkey agar plates that were incubated and observed for typical colonies of *P. aeruginosa.*

By far the most frequently employed medium for the determination of dilution counts is the liquid medium 10 of Drake (11). Inoculated tubes of Drake's medium are incubated at 38 to 39°C for up to 4 days. Cultures are examined daily for fluorescence under ultraviolet light. Cells from tubes exhibiting fluorescence are tested for their ability to utilize acetamide as the sole source of carbon and energy. Fluorescent pseudomonads that are capable of growth at 41°C but differ from *P. aeruginosa* often occur in certain wastes and in organically enriched surface waters when water temperatures approach 30°C (see following section). Such strains can produce reactions resembling those of *P. aeruginosa,* causing excessively high counts of *P. aeruginosa* in waters rich in organic matter when temperatures near 30°C (21; M. A. Levin, *personal communication*). Hoadley et al. (26) therefore added pyocyanin production on slants of King's A medium to confirm the presence of *P. aeruginosa.*

Robinton and Burk (53) compared recoveries of *P.*

aeruginosa from samples of river waters in Drake's medium and Trypticase Soy broth at 42°C. After incubation, each medium was streaked on MacConkey agar and on the cetrimide agar of Brown and Lowbury (6). Representative colonies were picked and their identity as *P. aeruginosa* confirmed by selected tests. *Pseudomonas aeruginosa* was isolated most frequently from MacConkey agar plates that were streaked from enrichments in Trypticase Soy broth. Mossel and Indacochea (45) employed enrichment in a rich peptone medium containing crystal violet, kanamycin, and tylosin, followed by streaking on a modified cetrimide medium of Brown and Lowbury (6) [glycerol−mannitol−acetamide−cetrimide (GMAC) agar] that contained acetamide and phenol red indicator, with mannitol replacing half the glycerol. The medium was incubated at 42°C, and colonies surrounded by red zones were counted. Recoveries of *P. aeruginosa* from sewage and lake water were slightly higher when this procedure was employed than when an earlier version of Drake's medium was employed.

Recently, several authors have reported successful isolation of *P. aeruginosa* from *Salmonella* enrichment broth. Gundstrup (20) observed that salmonellae and *P. aeruginosa* grew simultaneously in tetrathionate enrichment broth. Grunnet et al. (19) reported optimal recovery of *P. aeruginosa* from sewage in tetrathionate broth incubated for 2 to 4 days at 42°C and streaked on cetrimide agar that in turn was incubated at 42°C. Earlier, Némedi and Lányi (47) employed brilliant green selenite broth incubated at 37°C for 48 hr and streaked on brilliant green agar plates that in turn were incubated at 42°C for 24 hr to enumerate *P. aeruginosa* in raw and finished waters, swimming waters, and sewage. Similarly, Kenner (31,32) reported successful recovery of *P. aeruginosa* from sewage, sewage sludge, and potable water in dulcitol selenite broth incubated at 40°C for 24 to 48 hr and streaked on xylose lysine desoxycholate (XLD) agar which was incubated at 37°C for 24 hr.

Selenka (54) employed a medium containing 0.2% triphenyltetrazolium chloride for direct plating of sewage and polluted waters. Red colonies exhibiting positive cytochrome oxidase reactions were examined using selected tests to confirm their identity as *P. aeruginosa*. Selenka reported that two-thirds of the cytochrome oxidase positive colonies appearing on plates inoculated with river water were *P. aeruginosa*. Hoadley and McCoy (24), however, reported formation of colonies by only about 25% of cells of a *P. aeruginosa* test strain inoculated on Selenka's medium. Furthermore, the use of selective plating media, such as the solid medium of Drake (11) that contains 10^{-3}M cadmium chloride or the cetrimide agar of Brown and Lowbury (6), for the enumeration of *P. aeruginosa* in surface waters may lead to erroneous counts, as some cells that are injured during suspension may not form colonies (23). However, Mossel and Indacochea (45) reported counts of *P. aeruginosa* in sewage and lake water plated directly onto GMAC agar that were almost as high as dilution counts obtained with an earlier version of Drake's liquid medium.

Several media have been developed for use with membrane filters. The first, developed by Drake (11), contained 0.05% hexadecyltrimethyl ammonium bromide to inhibit growth of unwanted species. More recently, Levin and Cabelli (39) proposed a medium that contained sulfapyridine, kanamycin, nalidixic acid, and actidione in addition to indicator systems by which to recognize lactose, sucrose, and xylose fermenters and H_2S producers. Recoveries of *P. aeruginosa* cells stressed by suspension for up to 24 hr in estuarine water held at 6°C remained at approximately 90%.

Brodsky and Nixon (5) employed nonfluorescent black membrane filters to enumerate *P. aeruginosa* in swimming pool waters. Filters were incubated at 42°C for 24 hr on MacConkey agar plates. Following incubation, plates were allowed to stand at room temperature to permit development of fluorescence. Fluorescent colonies were counted under an ultraviolet light. Lantos et al. (35) incubated membrane filters on endoperoxidase (ENDO) agar for 24 and 48 hr at 37°C. Colonies were streaked on nutrient agar and deoxycholate citrate agar plates, and typical colonies were subsequently subjected to selected diagnostic tests.

MPNs of *P. aeruginosa* reported in this chapter were determined in Drake's medium 10 (11) incubated at 39°C up to 96 hr. Broth from fluorescent tubes was inoculated onto slants of acetamide agar and incubated as described previously (26). Cells from positive acetamide slants were inoculated onto slants of King's A medium (33) incubated at 30°C and observed daily up to 7 days for pyocyanin production. Only those tubes yielding pyocyanogenic *P. aeruginosa* were considered positive. Five tube MPNs were determined from tables (1).

CHARACTERISTICS OF STRAINS FROM SURFACE WATERS

Fluorescent pseudomonads that are capable of growth at 41°C can be isolated readily from most surface waters, particularly during warmer months. Generally, less than

10% of these fluorescent pseudomonads recovered from unpolluted or mildly polluted surface waters can be identified definitely as *P. aeruginosa* (21). Hoadley and Ajello (21) employed a series of 12 tests to distinguish *P. aeruginosa* from other strains of gram-negative rod-shaped bacteria that possess polar flagella, are able to grow at 41°C, exhibit oxidative glucose metabolism and a positive oxidase reaction, and produce fluorescent pigment on King's B medium incubated at 30°C (Table 1). Both pyocyanogenic and apyocyanogenic strains of *P. aeruginosa* exhibited little variability, and the species could be identified easily by these selected tests. Like *P. aeruginosa,* most questionable strains possessed a single polar flagellum and utilized geraniol, but they differed frequently with respect to hemolysis of human blood, liquefaction of gelatin, denitrification and utilization of mannitol and gluconate; the remaining tests provided important supportive evidence for differentiation. We agree with Sutter's conclusion (60) that fluorescent pseudomonads isolated from human carriers, clinical materials, and environmental sources, and which grow at 41°C but fail to denitrify or liquefy gelatin, probably are not *P. aeruginosa.*

Strains exhibiting reactions characteristic of *P. aeruginosa* usually can be subspeciated by immunotyping or pyocin typing and produce characteristic antibiograms. Strains that exhibit reactions differing from the characteristic pattern of *P. aeruginosa* are not typable by any of the above methods. Examination of a limited number of these strains indicates that they differ also in their cellular fatty acid compositions, which resemble those of the stutzeri and alcaligenes groups rather than the fluorescent group (C. W. Moss, *personal communi-*

TABLE 1. *Selected tests employed to distinguish* P. aeruginosa *from other fluorescent pseudomonads capable of growth at 41°C*

Test	Characteristic reaction of P. aeruginosa
No. of flagella	1
Pigment production	
Phenazine	+
Carotenoid	−
Hemolysis of human blood	+
Gelatin liquefaction	+
Denitrification	+
Utilization of	
Sebacate	+
Saccharate	−
Mannitol	+
Glycollate	−
Gluconate	+
Geraniol	+
Acetamide	+

cation). Although *P. aeruginosa* strains isolated during studies of surface waters not heavily polluted by hospital wastes were always susceptible to gentamicin and carbenicillin and were almost always resistant to chloramphenicol, streptomycin, tetracycline, neomycin, and kanamycin, strains differing from *P. aeruginosa* tended to be resistant to carbenicillin and susceptible to streptomycin and kanamycin (Table 2). Similarly, Blazevic et al. (4) noted that strains of *P. fluorescens* and *P. putida* were susceptible to kanamycin and resistant to carbenicillin, in contrast to resistance to kanamycin and susceptibility to carbenicillin exhibited by strains of *P. aeruginosa*. They suggested that susceptibility to these antibiotics would provide a rapid means of separating *P.*

TABLE 2. *Frequencies of fluorescent pseudomonads resistant to 7 antibiotics[a]*

Antibiotic	P. aeruginosa (35 strains)	Non-P. aeruginosa strains			
		Swimming pools (16 strains)	Polluted stream (21 strains)	Surface waters in Georgia (6 strains)	Surface waters in Georgia (9 strains)
Gentamicin	S[b](0)[c]	S(0)	S(0)	S(0)	S(0)
Carbenicillin	S(0)	R(16)	V(16)	S(0)	R(9)
Chloramphenicol	R(34)	R(16)	V(15)	V(2)	R(7/8)
Streptomycin	R(34)	S(0)	S(1)	S(0)	V(3)
Tetracycline	R(35)	R(16)	V(17)	S(0)	R(8)
Neomycin	R(33)	V(4)	V(11)	—	—
Kanamycin	R(34)	S(0)	S(0)	S(0)	S(0)

[a] Determined by the method of Bauer et al. (2). Resistant strains include strains exhibiting intermediate zones of inhibition. (Data from G. Ajello, D. Mooney, and A. W. Hoadley, *unpublished.*)
[b] S, susceptible; V, variable; R, resistant; —, not determined.
[c] Number of resistant strains.

aeruginosa from the other species in the clinical laboratory.

Pseudomonas strains selected for study were obtained from slants of King's A medium (33). Cells from the surface of King's A slants were transferred to Erlenmeyer flasks containing sterile nutrient broth and incubated overnight at room temperature on a rotary shaker. Appropriate dilutions were spread on plates of Trypticase Soy agar (Baltimore Biological Laboratories, Inc.) incubated overnight at 37°C. In some cases, cells from Drake's medium 10 or King's A slants were streaked directly on Drake's solid medium containing cadmium chloride (11) or on cetrimide agar (6), and were also incubated at 37°C. Isolated colonies were picked to nutrient agar slants to await study.

All strains reported possessed polar flagella, exhibited oxidative glucose metabolism, were oxidase positive, and produced fluorescent pigment on King's B medium (33). Other tests listed in Table 1 were performed as described by Hoadley and Ajello (21). Strains considered to differ from *P. aeruginosa* failed to denitrify and to hemolyse human blood, or they produced only a weak reaction on blood and commonly were unable to utilize mannitol and gluconate. In unpublished preliminary studies, no strain exhibiting these differences from the expected characteristics of *P. aeruginosa* thus far has been shown to produce pyocins detectable using the 18 indicator strains of Jones et al. (30); nor have any strains been typable by either the Parke-Davis or Difco antisera.

Immunotyping was performed with seven antisera (16) provided by H. B. Devlin (Parke-Davis and Co.) according to accompanying instructions. Susceptibility to seven antibiotics was determined by the method of Bauer et al.

(2). Antibiotics included tetracycline (30 μg), chloramphenicol (30 μg), streptomycin (10 μg), kanamycin (30 μg), neomycin (30 μg), gentamicin (10 μg), and carbenicillin (100 μg). Results were recorded as susceptible or resistant. Strains exhibiting zones of inhibition falling in the intermediate category were classified as resistant.

POPULATIONS IN SURFACE WATERS

Although *P. aeruginosa* may, under appropriate conditions, occur naturally in surface waters, the species probably does not normally inhabit northern temperature surface waters unless recently affected by human activity or the activities of domestic animals (27). It is probable that *P. aeruginosa* is associated primarily with man. Although the incidence of intestinal carriage has been reported to vary in different countries, the rate in the United States (Table 3) appears to be slightly in excess of 10% among healthy adults (26,43,52,61) and increases among certain hospitalized patients (29,40,58,59). Fecal carriage in domestic animals appears to occur primarily as a result of contact with human carriers (25).

The major potential source of *P. aeruginosa* in surface waters is domestic sewage (26). Populations in excess of 10^5/100 ml are common, although populations in excess of 10^6/100 ml have been demonstrated in raw sewage in Germany (55). Storm drainage and barnyard runoff may act as lesser sources (Table 4). Furthermore, slaughterhouse wastes may contain large numbers of *P. aeruginosa* and constitute a potential source if they are released directly into the environment. Populations of *P. aeruginosa* in hospital wastes frequently exceed 10^6/100 ml (17; A. W. Hoadley, *unpublished data*). However,

TABLE 3. *Frequency of isolation of* P. aeruginosa *from feces and rectal swabs of healthy adults in the United States*

No. examined	No. positive	% positive	Reference
103	16	15.6	29
100	11	11	52
273	32	11.7	43
235	28	11.9	61
52	6	11.5	26
104[a]	13	12.5	58

[a] Reconstructive patients in good health in a burns institute for children.

TABLE 4. *Sources of* P. aeruginosa *in surface waters* [a]

Source	Median MPN/100 ml
Sewage (Madison, Wisc.)	
Raw	2.25×10^5
After treatment	3.5×10^3
Meat packing wastes	
After treatment	2.9×10^5
Storm drainage	
(Madison, Wisc.)	2.9×10^2
Barnyard runoff	7.8×10^0

[a] From A. W. Hoadley et al., ref. 26.

hospital wastes are of special concern only if they are discharged directly without treatment, or with inadequate treatment. On the other hand, bacterial strains in hospital wastes discharged to streams may be of special interest because they can bear resistance to certain antibiotics. In recent years, *P. aeruginosa* strains resistant to carbenicillin and to gentamicin have appeared in hospitals. While strains isolated from hospital wastes appear not to be resistant to gentamicin, carbenicillin-resistant strains have been demonstrated in both hospital wastes and polluted stream waters (Table 5).

Populations of *P. aeruginosa* in surface waters receiving low but definite levels of contamination may vary from 1 to 10 *P. aeruginosa*/100 ml (11,27,55). Populations exceeding 100 bacteria/100 ml, but less than 1,000/100 ml were demonstrated in earlier investigations of polluted streams (24,54). More recently, however, Hoadley et al. (27) demonstrated median populations of between 1,300 and 9,500 *P. aeruginosa*/100 ml downstream from unchlorinated settled sewage outfalls. In the latter studies, populations were observed to decrease by more than 90% within 3 hr, but the rate of decrease increased greatly with the temperature of the water (Fig. 1). Studies undertaken in southern waters indicate that higher populations may be encountered in streams below hospital waste discharges and that the bacteria may influence streams for several miles downstream (Table 6).

Organically enriched surface waters are capable of supporting growth of *P. aeruginosa* in the laboratory,

TABLE 5. *Occurrence of* P. aeruginosa *isolates resistant to carbenicillin[a] in hospital wastes and a receiving stream[b]*

Source of isolates	No. tested	No. resistant	% resistant
Stream above outfall	35	0	0
Hospital wastes	109	20	12.0
Stream below outfall	186	24	18.4

[a] Resistance determined by the method of Bauer et al. (2) with 100 μg discs.
[b] Data from A. W. Hoadley and G. Ajello, *unpublished.*

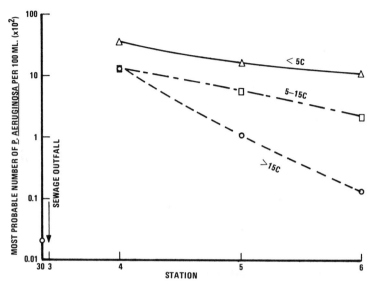

FIG. 1. Median MPNs of *P. aeruginosa* in a stream in Wisconsin receiving unchlorinated primary sewage. (From Hoadley et al., ref. 27.)

and Hoadley et al. (27) suggested that, on the basis of this observation and the occasional recovery of the species from unpolluted but organically enriched surface waters when water temperatures exceeded 30°C, growth might occur when the temperatures were high. Although such temperatures are rare in the northern United States, they are not uncommon in the southern part of the country, and a direct relationship between water temperature and *P. aeruginosa* populations has been demonstrated (21). *Pseudomonas aeruginosa* was isolated from cold waters only following rains, which suggested that soil may constitute a reservoir of the bacteria that reaches surface waters. Similar data are reported in Table 7. The increas-

TABLE 6. *Most probable numbers of* P. aeruginosa *in a stream receiving hospital wastes*[a]

Station	Distance below outfall (mi)	Time of flow(min)	Flow (cfs)	Median MPN/100 ml
1 (upstream)	—	—	—	4.7×10^2
2 (at outfall)[b]	0	0	5.53	5.7×10^3
3	0.55	50	6.74	1.8×10^4
4	1.0	99	7.11	9.0×10^3
5	1.85	183	8.89	3.1×10^2
6	2.45	ND[c]	ND	3.3×10

[a] Data from D. Mooney and A. W. Hoadley, *unpublished.*
[b] Waste not well mixed with stream water.
[c] Not determinable.

ingly frequent isolations and the increasing numbers suggest that growth occurs in unpolluted, but organically rich, waters as the temperatures increase. Decreases in populations that occur in waters at higher temperatures probably are a result of the rapid death of bacteria caused by increased metabolism and predation rates.

The frequencies of immunotypes among *P. aeruginosa* strains isolated from surface waters resembled in some respects frequencies reported from hospitalized patients, but differed significantly from others. Frequencies encountered among strains from unpolluted or remotely polluted surface waters and from stream waters receiving hospital wastes are presented in Table 8. The incidences of type 1 strains in both polluted and unpolluted waters were similar to those reported among 742 strains isolated from hospitalized patients by Moody et al. (44). On the other hand, although less than 1% of strains examined by Moody were untypable, approximately 20% of all strains

TABLE 7. *Occurrence of P. aeruginosa in surface waters of north central Georgia*[a]

Water source	Temperature of water (°C)	Total no. of samples	No. positive	% positive	MPN/100 ml Median	MPN/100 ml Range
Unpolluted	≤ 15	32	11	34.4	< 1.8	< 1.8–13
	15–30	23	10	43.5	< 1.8	< 1.8–7.8
	≥ 30	13	10	76.9	4.5	< 1.8–49
Remote fecal pollution	≤ 15	20	15	75.0	1.8	< 1.8–40
	15–30	65	39	60.0	1.8	< 1.8–180
	≥ 30	22	10	45.4	< 1.8	< 1.8–17

[a] Data from D. E. Knight and A. W. Hoadley, *unpublished*; and from A. W. Hoadley and G. Ajello, ref. 21.

TABLE 8. *Frequencies of* P. aeruginosa *immunotypes among isolates from surface waters*[a]

Parke-Davis immunotype	Lake waters (288 strains)	Polluted stream (214 strains)
1	37.5[b]	28.1
2	5.9	13.1
3	2.8	4.2
4	8.7	9.3
5	1.7	0.7
6	2.1	1.4
7	6.2	10.3
3,7	5.6	10.3
Other strong cross reactions	4.9	1.4
Rough	1.4	3.7
Untypable	23.2	17.3

[a] Data from G. Ajello, D. Mooney, and A. W. Hoadley, *unpublished.*
[b] Percent of strains.

from surface waters were untypable by the seven antisera of Parke-Davis and Co. Also, types 3, 5, and 6 were encountered less frequently among isolates from surface waters than among clinical isolates (10.5, 6.6, and 19.9%, respectively). Type 4 was encountered more frequently, in approximately 9% of isolates from surface waters, as compared to 4.6% of isolates from clinical sources. Lanyi et al. (37) and Némedi and Lányi (47) recognized a striking similarity of *P. aeruginosa* serotypes in water samples from numerous sources, including sewage and human feces, employing 13 antisera according to Lányi (36).

OCCURRENCE IN DRINKING WATERS

Pseudomonas aeruginosa may be isolated from finished drinking water supplies. Hunter and Ensign (29) isolated the species from 4 of 72 private wells. Grieble et al. (18) recommended that chlorinated tap water not be used in humidifier reservoirs because it supported luxuriant growth of *Pseudomonas*. On the other hand, Edmondson et al. (12) recommended the use of chlorinated tap water in nebulizer jars because it retarded multiplication of *P. aeruginosa*. As a rule, *P. aeruginosa* seldom can be isolated from drinking waters, especially treated drinking waters, unless fecal contamination or some other source of the organism exists (Table 9). Contamination of the Szeged waters (35) occurred as a result of infiltration of sewage into underground storage basins.

TABLE 9. *Occurrence of* P. aeruginosa *in drinking water samples*

Source of samples	No. of samples	No. positive	% positive	Refer- ence
Water supplies in northern Israel	1,000	241	24.1	51
Water supplies in Hungary				
Satisfactory well supplies	2,774	31	1.1	37
spring supplies	123	4	3.3	37
finished waters	2,785	10	0.4	37
Unsatisfactory well supplies	2,519	54	2.1	37
spring supplies	47	3	6.4	37
finished waters	971	14	1.4	37
Budapest municipal supply				
membrane filter	34,429	88	0.2	37
most probable number	353	12	3.4	37
Szeged uncontaminated finished waters	374	6	1.6	36
contaminated finished waters	133	46	34.5	36
Finished waters in southern Ontario	14,486	57	0.4	8

The relatively frequent demonstration of *P. aeruginosa* reported by Reitler and Seligmann (51) for northern Israel water supplies may be related to the character of the waters or to the use of more effective isolation techniques. There was no relationship between coliform counts and counts of *P. aeruginosa*. Kenner and Clark (31) reported the isolation of *P. aeruginosa* from 17 of 20 samples from water supplies in the United States, including wells, cisterns, and small municipal supplies. Fecal coliforms were not detected in most supplies investigated, although fecal streptococci were detected in some.

Hoadley and Cheng (23) reported that *P. aeruginosa* cells suspended in Atlanta tap water underwent injury that prevented recovery on the highly selective solid medium of Drake (11) and caused a rapid decline in the viable count determined on Trypticase Soy agar (Fig. 2). The tap waters employed in these studies were free of residual chlorine when taken from the tap. Samples were removed periodically from tap water inoculated with *P. aeruginosa* and placed on Trypticase Soy agar and Drake's medium. Thus, tap waters may be toxic to cells of *P. aeruginosa,* which tends to support the majority of published findings. On the other hand, in view of the demonstration by Favero et al. (14) of growth after 48 hr in distilled water of *P. aeruginosa* grown initially in a rich medium, the possibility of growth following an initial period of decline in some nontoxic finished drinking waters cannot be excluded.

WATER AS A VEHICLE FOR TRANSMISSION

Although it is known that surface waters may carry *P. aeruginosa* to plants, animals, and man, the significance

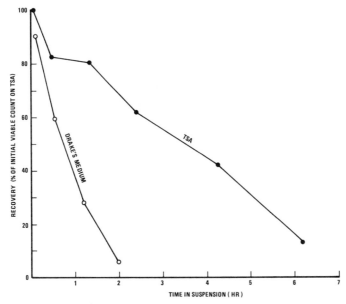

FIG. 2. Recovery of *P. aeruginosa* ATCC 10145 from tap water. (From Hoadley and Cheng, ref. 23.)

of contaminated surface waters as vehicles for the transmission of strains causing disease in man is not understood. Drinking waters rarely carry *P. aeruginosa* and often are toxic to the organism. However, some drinking waters, if grossly contaminated, may at times transmit the bacteria. Populations develop naturally in organically enriched surface waters when water temperatures approach or exceed 30°C, or may originate from soil in warm climates; but the major sources of the species in water are wastes from man and from animals closely associated with man. If the application of sewage and sewage sludge to the land increases in response to rising costs of fertilizer, the opportunity for the spread to plants and for the contamination of surface waters may be increased.

Our knowledge of the ecology of *P. aeruginosa* in surface waters is limited, however, and we know little of the serotypes that grow or survive well in the environment, routes by which the organism may spread, or even the classification and significance of apyocyanogenic fluorescent pseudomonads resembling *P. aeruginosa*. A greater understanding of these matters must be achieved before we can know the importance of surface waters in the transmission of *P. aeruginosa*.

REFERENCES

1. American Public Health Association (1971): Standard methods for the examination of water and wastewater. 13th ed. American Public Health Association, Inc., New York.
2. Bauer, A. W., Kirby, W. M., Sherris, J. C., and Turck, M. (1966): Antibiotic susceptibility testing by a standardized single disc method. *Am. J. Clin. Pathol.*, 45:493–496.
3. Bechenhauer, W. H., and Miner, C. A. (1960): *Pseudomonas* infection in mink. *Vet. Rec.*, 55:55–56.
4. Blazevic, D. J., Koepcke, M. H., and Matsen, J. M. (1973): Incidence and identification of *Pseudomonas fluorescens* and *Pseudomonas putida* in the clinical laboratory. *Appl. Microbiol.*, 25:107–110.
5. Brodsky, M. H., and Nixon, M. C. (1974): Membrane filter method for the isolation and enumeration of *Pseudomonas aeruginosa* from swimming pools. *Appl. Microbiol.*, 27:938–943.
6. Brown, V. I., and Lowbury, E. J. L. (1965): Use of an improved cetrimide agar medium and other culture methods for *Pseudomonas aeruginosa*. *J. Clin. Pathol.*, 18:752–756.
7. Cherrington, V. A., and Gildow, E. M. (1931): Bovine mastitis caused by *Pseudomonas aeruginosa*. *J. Am. Vet. Med. Assoc.*, 79:803–808.
8. Clark, J. A., and Vlassoff, L. T. (1973): Relationships among pollution indicator bacteria isolated from raw water and distribution systems by the presence-absence (P–A) test. *Health Lab. Sci.*, 10:163–172.

9. Cothran, W. W., and Hatlen, J. B. (1962): A study of an outdoor swimming pool using iodine for water disinfection. *Stud. Med.*, 10:493–502.
10. Curtis, P. E. (1969): *Pseudomonas aeruginosa* contamination of a warm water system used for pre-milking udder washing. *Vet. Rec.*, 84:476–477.
11. Drake, C. H. (1966): Evaluation of culture media for the isolation and enumeration of *Pseudomonas aeruginosa. Health Lab. Sci.*, 3:10–19.
12. Edmondson, E. B., Rainarz, J. A., Pierce, A. K., and Sanford, J. P. (1966): Nebulization equipment: A potential source of infection in Gram-negative pneumonias. *Am. J. Dis. Child.*, 111:357–360.
13. Elrod, R. P., and Brown, A. C. (1942): *Pseudomonas aeruginosa:* Its role as a plant pathogen. *J. Bacteriol.*, 44:633–645.
14. Favero, M. S., Carson, L. A., Bond, W. W., and Petersen, N. J. (1971): *Pseudomonas aeruginosa:* Growth in distilled water from hospitals. *Science,* 173:836–838.
15. Favero, M. S., Drake, C. H., and Randall, G. B., (1964): Use of staphylococci as indicators of swimming pool pollution. *U.S. Publ. Health Rep.*, 79:61–70.
16. Fisher, N. W., Devlin, H. B., and Gnabasik, F. J. (1969): New immunotype scheme for *Pseudomonas aeruginosa* based on protective antigens. *J. Bacteriol.*, 98:835–836.
17. Grabow, W. O. K., and Nupen, E. M. (1972): The load of infectious microorganisms in the waste water of two South African hospitals. *Water Res.*, 6:1557–1563.
18. Grieble, H. G., Colton, F. R., Bird, T. J., Toigo, A., and Griffith, L. G. (1970): Fine-particle humidifiers: Source of *Pseudomonas aeruginosa* infections in a respiratory-disease unit. *N. Engl. J. Med.*, 282:531–535.
19. Grunnet, K., Gundstrup, A. S. P., and Bonde, G. J. (1974): Tetrathionate broth as a medium for simultaneous demonstration of *Salmonella* and *Pseudomonas aeruginosa. Nord. Vet. Med.*, 26:239–242.
20. Gundstrup, A. S. P. (1974): Competitive growth of *Salmonella* and pseudomonads in tetrathionate enrichment broth. *Health Lab. Sci.*, 11:25–27.
21. Hoadley, A. W., and Ajello, G. (1972): Some characteristics of fluorescent pseudomonads isolated from surface waters and capable of growth at 41C. *Can. J. Microbiol.*, 18:1769–1773.
22. Hoadley, A. W., Ajello, G., and Masterson, N. (1975): Preliminary studies of fluorescent pseudomonads capable of growth at

41C in swimming pool waters. *Appl. Microbiol.,* 29:527–531.

23. Hoadley, A. W., and Cheng, C. M. (1974): The recovery of indicator bacteria on selective media. *J. Appl. Bacteriol.,* 37:45–57.

24. Hoadley, A. W., and McCoy, E. (1966): Studies of certain Gram-negative bacteria from surface waters. *Health Lab. Sci.,* 3:20–32.

25. Hoadley, A. W., and McCoy, E. (1968): Some observations on the ecology of *Pseudomonas aeruginosa* and its occurrence in the intestinal tracts of animals. *Cornell Vet.,* 58:354–363.

26. Hoadley, A. W., McCoy, E., and Rohlich, G. A. (1968): Untersuchungen uber *Pseudomonas aeruginosa* in Oberflachengewassern. I. Quellen. *Arch. Hyg. Bakteriol.,* 152:328–338.

27. Hoadley, A. W., McCoy, E., and Rohlich, G. A. (1968): Untersuchungen uber *Pseudomonas aeruginosa* in Oberflachengewassern. II. Auftreten und Verhalten. *Arch. Hyg. Bakteriol.,* 152:339–344.

28. Hoitink, H. A. J., Hagedorn, D. J., and McCoy, E. (1968): Survival, transmission and taxonomy of *Pseudomonas syringae* van Hall, the causal organism of bacterial brown spot of bean (*Phaseolus vulgaris* L.). *Can J. Microbiol.,* 14:437–441.

29. Hunter, C. A., and Ensign, P. R. (1947): An epidemic of diarrhea in a newborn nursery caused by *Pseudomonas aeruginosa. Am. J. Publ. Health,* 37:1166–1169.

30. Jones, L. F., Zakanycz, J. P., Thomas, E. T., and Farmer III, J. J. (1974): Pyocin typing of *Pseudomonas aeruginosa:* A simplified method. *Appl. Microbiol.,* 27:400–406.

31. Kenner, B. A., and Clark, H. P. (1974): Detection and enumeration of *Salmonella* and *Pseudomonas aeruginosa. J. Water Pollut. Control Fed.,* 46:2163–2171.

32. Kenner, B. A., Dotson, G. K., and Smith, J. E. (1971): Simultaneous quantitation of *Salmonella* species and *Pseudomonas aeruginosa.* National Environmental Research Center, U. S. Environmental Protection Agency, Cincinnati.

33. King, E. O., Ward, M. K., and Raney, D. E. (1954): Two single media for the demonstration of pyocyanin and fluorescin. *J. Lab. Clin. Med.,* 44:301–307.

34. Kominos, S. D., Copeland, C. E., Grosiak, B., and Postic, B. (1972): Introduction of *Pseudomonas aeruginosa* into a hospital via vegetables. *Appl. Microbiol.,* 24:567–570.

35. Lantos, J., Kiss, M., Lányi, B., and Völgyesi, J. (1969): Serological and phage typing of *Pseudomonas aeruginosa* invading a municipal water supply. *Acta Microbiol. Acad. Sci. Hung.,* 16:333–336.

36. Lányi, B. (1966): Serological properties of *Pseudomonas aeruginosa*. I. Group-specific somatic antigens. *Acta Microbiol. Acad. Sci. Hung.*, 13:295–318.
37. Lányi, B., Gregacs, M., and Ádám, M. M. (1966): Incidence of *Pseudomonas aeruginosa* serogroups in water and human faeces. *Acta Microbiol. Acad. Sci. Hung.*, 13:319–326.
38. Larrivee, G. P., and Elvehjem, C. A. (1954): Disease problems in chinchillas. *J. Am. Vet. Med. Assoc.*, 124:447–455.
39. Levin, M. A., and Cabelli, V. J. (1972): Membrane filter technique for enumeration of *Pseudomonas aeruginosa*. *Appl. Microbiol.*, 24:864–870.
40. Lowbury, E. J. L., and Fox, J. (1954): The epidemiology of infection with *Pseudomonas pyocyanea* in a burns unit. *J. Hyg.*, 52:403–416.
41. Malmo, J., Robinson, B., and Morris, R. S. (1972): An outbreak of mastitis due to *Pseudomonas aeruginosa* in a dairy herd. *Am. Vet. J.*, 48:137–139.
42. McDonald, R. A., and Pinheiro, A. F. (1967): Water chlorination controls *Pseudomonas aeruginosa* in a rabbitry. *J. Am. Vet. Med. Assoc.*, 151:863–864.
43. Mills, G. Y., and Kagan, B. M. (1954): Effects of oral polymyxin B on *Pseudomonas aeruginosa* in the gastrointestinal tract. *Ann. Intern. Med.*, 40:26–32.
44. Moody, M. R., Young, V. M., Kenton, D. M., and Vermeulen, G. D. (1972): *Pseudomonas aeruginosa* in a center for cancer research. I. Distribution of intraspecies types from human and environmental sources. *J. Infect. Dis.*, 125:95–101.
45. Mossel, D. A. A., and Indacochea, L. (1971): A new cetrimide medium for the detection of *Pseudomonas aeruginosa*. *J. Med. Microbiol.*, 4:380–382.
46. Mushin, R., and Ziv, G. (1973): An epidemiological study of *Pseudomonas aeruginosa* in cattle and other animals by pyocine typing. *J. Hyg.*, 71:113–122.
47. Némedi, L., and Lányi, B. (1971): Incidence and hygienic importance of *Pseudomonas aeruginosa* in water. *Acta Microbiol. Acad. Sci. Hung.*, 18:319–326.
48. Pickens, E. M., Welsh, M. F., and Poelma, L. J. (1926): Pyocyaneus bacillosis and mastitis due to *Ps. aeruginosa*. *Cornell Vet.*, 16:186–202.
49. Prassad, B. M., Srivastava, C. P., Narayan, K. G., and Prasad, A. K. (1968): Source of *Pseudomonas* infection in calves. *Indian J. Anim. Health*, 7:51–54.
50. Radaelli, G., and Perini, G. (1960): Contributo allo studia della

mastite bovina da *"Pseudomonas aeruginosa." Arch. Vet. Ital.*, 11:294.

51. Reitler, R., and Seligmann, R. (1957): *Pseudomonas aeruginosa* in drinking water. *J. Appl. Bacteriol.*, 20:145–150.
52. Ringen, L. M., and Drake, C. H. (1952): A study of the incidence of *Pseudomonas aeruginosa* from various natural sources. *J. Bacteriol.*, 64:841–845.
53. Robinton, E. D., and Burk, C. J. (1972): The Mill River and its floodplain in Northampton and Williamsburg, Massachusetts: A study of the vascular plant flora, vegetation, and the presence of the bacterial family *Pseudomonadaceae* in relation to patterns of land use. Water Resources Research Center, Univ. of Massachusetts. Completion Report 72–4.
54. Selenka, F. (1960): Der quantitative Nachweis von *Pseudomonas aeruginosa* in Oberflachenwasser. *Arch. Hyg. Bakteriol.*, 144:627–634.
55. Selenka, F., and Ruschke, R. (1965): Keimzahlen und Fakalindikatoren in Bodenseewasser. *Arch. Hyg. Bakteriol.*, 149:273–287.
56. Shooter, R. A., Cooke, E. M., Faiers, M. C., Breaden, A. L., and O'Farrel, S. M. (1971): Isolation of *Escherichia coli, Pseudomonas aeruginosa,* and *Klebsiella* from food in hospitals, canteens, and schools. *Lancet,* 2:390–392.
57. Shooter, R. A., Cooke, E. M., Gaya, H., Kumar, P., Patel, N., Parker, M. T., Thom, B. T., and Grance, D. R. (1969): Food and medicaments as possible sources of hospital strains of *Pseudomonas aeruginosa. Lancet,* 1:1227–1229.
58. Smith, R. F., Dayton, S. L., Chipps, D. D., and Blasi, D. (1973): Intestinal carriage of *Klebsiella* and *Pseudomonas* in burned children and their comparative role in nosocomial infection. *Health Lab. Sci.,* 10:173–179.
59. Stoodley, B. J., and Thom, B. T. (1970): Observations on the intestinal carriage of *Pseudomonas aeruginosa. J. Med. Microbiol.,* 3:367–375.
60. Sutter, V. L. (1968): Identification of *Pseudomonas* species isolated from hospital environment and human sources. *Appl. Microbiol.,* 16:1532–1538.
61. Sutter, V. L., Hurst, V., and Lane, C. W. (1967): Quantification of *Pseudomonas aeruginosa* in feces of healthy human adults. *Health Lab. Sci.,* 4:245–249.
62. Taplin, D., and Mertz, P. M. Flower vases in hospitals as reservoirs of pathogens. *Lancet,* 2:1279–1281.

63. Thomas, M. E. M., Piper, E., and Maurer, I. M. (1972): Contamination of an operating theater by Gram-negative bacteria. Examination of water supplies, cleaning methods and wound infections. *J. Hyg.,* 70:63–73.
64. Trautwein, G., Helmboldt, C. F., and Nielsen, S. W. (1962): Pathology of *Pseudomonas* pneumonia in mink. *J. Am. Vet. Med. Assoc.,* 140:701–704.
65. Weber, G., Werner, ,H. P., and Matschnigg, H. (1971): *Pseudomonas aeruginosa* in Trinkwasser als Todesursache bei Neugeborenen. *Zentralbl. Bakteriol. Parasitenk. Infektionskr. Hyg. I Abt. Orig.,* 216:210–214.

Pseudomonas aeruginosa: Ecological Aspects and Patient Colonization, edited by Viola Mae Young. Raven Press, New York © 1977.

Pseudomonas aeruginosa from Vegetables, Salads, and Other Foods Served to Patients with Burns

*Spyros D. Kominos, **Charles E. Copeland, and **Carol A. Delenko

*Microbiology Section and **Division of General Surgery, Mercy Hospital, Pittsburgh, Pennsylvania 15219*

Pseudomonas aeruginosa is not generally considered to be pathogenic to healthy humans, yet it has the capacity to cause common and severe infections in hospitalized patients with underlying primary disease. Alexander (1) recently reviewed *P. aeruginosa* as an emerging pathogen in debilitated patients, especially those with burn traumas. This author emphasized the use of antibiotics as a prime factor in the progressive shift of opportunistic pathogens in these patients from *Staphylococcus* and *Streptococcus* to gram-negative bacilli such as *P. aeruginosa*. Although *Pseudomonas* infection primarily manifests itself as wound sepsis or bacteremia, it is not unusual for this organism to cause urinary and respiratory tract infections. In burn wards where several patients are brought together, *Pseudomonas* outbreaks can be (a) sporadic, involving one, two or three patients with no

59

apparent common exposure, or (b) hyperendemic, when most or all patients are infected in generalized situations that can last for prolonged periods of time (10). Such hyperendemic infections can be catastrophic to patients and demoralizing to medical and nursing personnel.

HYPERENDEMIC SITUATION

From early 1970 to mid-1971 a hyperendemic situation existed in our burn center. Studies undertaken then showed that as many as four different types of *P. aeruginosa* could be recovered from the wounds of an individual patient and that several patients could share the same types at a particular point in time. This suggested cross-contamination among patients (5). About 20% of cultures from hands of nurses at that time were positive with types of *P. aeruginosa* identical to those recovered from patients. These findings would appear to indicate that direct handling of patients by nursing personnel was a principal mode of transmission (5). Lowbury and his associates (9) have also shown in a definitive study that such contact was a major means of *P. aeruginosa* transmission in wards with many susceptible patients.

CONTROL PROGRAM

In August 1971 a program to reduce environmental contamination in the center was initiated. Hand washing with an iodophore scrub was rigidly enforced and all personnel entering the room were required to wash their hands in a sink located by the entrance. Gowns were mandatory for all those entering the center. A new hy-

drotherapy tank that could be easily disinfected was installed for debridement of patients. Use of whirlpool motors
was discontinued because repeated efforts to decontami-
nate them had failed. The tank was washed with
povidone-iodine scrub and rinsed between patients; repeated cultures showed no evidence of contamination.
Other environmental cultures negative for *P. aeruginosa*
were from floors (after mopping), saline solutions, washing basins, suction tubes, medicated creams, and table
and counter surfaces. Occasionally, *P. aeruginosa* was
recovered from cultures of the sinks in the unit. The
nurses were instructed to consider sinks as potential
sources of infection and the housekeeping personnel
were asked to clean the sinks daily with Clorox; no at-
tempts, however, were made to sterilize them since previous studies had shown that direct infection of wounds
was not caused by types of *P. aeruginosa* previously
recovered from sinks (5,9). At the same time arrangements were made to sterilize all respiratory therapy
equipment such as tubing, nebulizers, humidifiers, res-
pirometers, and others. All these items were cultured
weekly to determine the level of contamination while in
use. The water in nebulizers and humidifiers was
changed every 8 hr.

RE-EVALUATION

After the environment in the burn center was found to
be free of *P. aeruginosa* (except for occasional positive
cultures from sinks) and the environmental control program was being observed, we expected the rate of infection to drop significantly. From August 1971 to September 1973 the pattern of infection did change favorably

from hyperendemic to sporadic outbreaks. The infection rate dropped from approximately 80 to 32% and remained at that rate for 2 years. During that time *Pseudomonas* infections would subside for several days and would reappear later, generally beginning with the severely burned patient, usually after the first week of their admission. It was also observed that several patients developed wound sepsis first in the perineal area and thighs, followed by wound infections on the legs, feet, abdomen, shoulders, chest, and arms. Because of the location of the primary wound sepsis, it was suspected that *P. aeruginosa* was excreted with stools and subsequently contaminated the wounds.

COLONIZATION OF THE GASTROINTESTINAL TRACT AND HOSPITAL ACQUISITION OF *P. AERUGINOSA*

Pseudomonas aeruginosa has been shown to be carried in the gastrointestinal tract by 3 to 6% of healthy individuals (8,13,18). Although Shooter and associates (16) found the organism in 24% of newly admitted patients, much higher recovery rates were found after prolonged hospitalization; it was isolated from stools of 43% of the patients receiving antibiotics and 53% of the gastrointestinal surgery patients (18).

During the time of our studies, Schimpff and his associates (12) reported that patients with acute lymphocytic leukemia developed *Pseudomonas* infections from their own flora. These authors found, however, that most patients became colonized (as shown by rectal swabs) after admission to the hospital. Since *Pseudomonas* infection of patients was commonly preceded by gastrointestinal colonization with the infecting strains, it was suggested "that a very large proportion of infections might be avoided if hospital acquisition of potential pathogens could be prevented."

How do patients acquire *P. aeruginosa* in the gastrointestinal tract after admission to the hospital? During sporadic outbreaks of *Pseudomonas* infections in our burn center, we noticed that each patient usually carried a different type of *P. aeruginosa*. Such individual rather than epidemic outbreaks had been observed earlier also by Shooter and his associates (14) who suspected them to be self-infections with *P. aeruginosa* from the patient's own flora, and they were able to demonstrate that food could contribute to intestinal colonization of patients. With these observations and questions in mind, we undertook studies to determine which foods served to our patients might contain this microorganism and how these foods could serve as reservoirs and vehicles of transmission for *P. aeruginosa*. Means and methods could then be established that would aid in the reduction and control of *P. aeruginosa*.

PATIENTS, THERAPY, AND CULTURES

The burn center is a seven-bed ward isolated from the rest of the hospital to minimize contamination of these high-risk patients. The ages of our patients range from infancy to 80 years old, with three-fourths of the patients being adults from 30 to 60 years old. Injuries extend from 5 to 60% of the body surface area and consist of both second- and third-degree burns.

Since 1970 the patients on admission have received antibiotics for 3 days (penicillin, 600,000 U q.i.d. and streptomycin, 500 mg t.i.d.). They also have received daily cleansing of the burn wounds in the hydrotherapy tank and application of povidone-iodine topical ointment. If *Pseudomonas* infection was suspected, it was confirmed by at least one of two methods: (a) the recovery of *P. aeruginosa* from biweekly surface cultures for at least 2 weeks or (b) quantitative cultures of eschar from which at least 10^5 *Pseudomonas*/g were recovered.

Salads and vegetable samples weighing from 50 to 200 g were obtained from the hospital kitchen. Most vegetables had been rinsed with tap water by kitchen personnel and set in large colanders until cut for salads; however, some were obtained directly from delivery trucks prior to contact with kitchen personnel. Individual salad portions were obtained from the kitchen prior to patient distribution.

Vegetables tested in this study were shipped from the South and the West and most commonly from Florida, Louisiana, and central California. No attempt was made to determine the relationship of geographical origin of the vegetables to the frequency of *P. aeruginosa* recovery.

All samples were cultured within 3 hr after collection. They were weighed and then homogenized for 60 sec in a sterile Waring blender. In order to facilitate homogenization, sterile distilled water was added in volumes equal to the weight of each sample of salads and vegetables except tomatoes. With the use of a glass rod, spread plates of the homogenate were prepared by plating 0.1 ml/plate on two plates of cetrimide agar (0.03% cetrimide in Mueller-Hinton agar, BBL). Two tubes of 5 ml acetamide broth (17) were inoculated with 0.5 ml homogenate.

All plates were incubated at 42°C and were examined with a Wood's lamp for fluorescence after 24 and 48 hr.

Final counts were taken when fluorescence was easily observed, usually at 24 hr. Broth cultures were incubated for 48 hr at 42°C, subcultured onto cetrimide agar, and incubated at 42°C for 24 hr before examination under the Wood's lamp.

Colonies on cetrimide agar with yellow-green or blue-green fluorescence under a Wood's lamp were suspected to be *P. aeruginosa*. For identification, in addition to growth on cetrimide agar at 42°C, fluorescence and pigment production, three other tests were performed on one to five colonies from each sample: oxidase, motility, and oxidation of glucose (4).

From each cetrimide plate three to five colonies of *P. aeruginosa* were pyocine typed; strains isolated from clinical specimens were also pyocin typed. In principle, a pyocin-producing isolate of *P. aeruginosa* is recognized as a certain type by the pattern of the inhibition produced against 11 indicator strains. The procedure used is presented in detail by Zabransky and Day (19).

Specimens from milkshakes and feeding formulas were obtained from the burn center and the kitchen. Samples of 10 ml were transferred to the laboratory and cultured on cetrimide agar (0.1 ml on each of two plates) and acetamide broth (0.5 ml into each of two tubes). Plates and tubes were incubated and treated by the same procedures as described previously for salads and vegetables.

RECOVERY OF *P. AERUGINOSA* FROM VEGETABLE SALADS, MILKSHAKES AND FEEDING FORMULAS

Shooter and his associates (14) found *P. aeruginosa* in foods from the hospital kitchen and in samples of medicine; they also recovered, from the feces of patients, strains of the organism that were similar to those carried in the substances ingested by the patients. Two years later the same group of investigators (15) reported that they found *P. aeruginosa* along with *Klebsiella* and *Escherichia coli* mostly in salads, milk feeds, and occasionally in cold and hot foods. These authors recommended that such foods, especially milk feeds, should be free of potentially pathogenic bacteria when given to susceptible patients, because they can lead to intestinal colonization. Although those investigators did not implicate fresh vegetables as the sources of *P. aeruginosa,* we decided to examine vegetable salads and whole vegetables as likely sources of bacterial transmission, since these foods were given uncooked and constituted part of the daily menu of many patients in our burn center.

As suspected, we isolated *P. aeruginosa* from vegetable salads (and from vegetables) and we reported the original results in October 1972 (6). Data accumulated subsequently confirming our early findings are presented here. In Table 1 it is shown that *P. aeruginosa* was recovered from 52 of 115 (45%) vegetable salad samples with almost half of the positive samples giving counts of 10^2 or more *Pseudomonas*/g. In addition, milkshakes and feeding formulas were examined and it was found that 6 of 10 milkshakes and 9 of 34 feeding formulas contained *P. aeruginosa*. Half-pint paper cartons of milk given to patients were cultured and found to be free of gram-negative bacteria. As a consequence, the Waring blenders used to make the milkshakes were cultured and *P. aeruginosa* was recovered 8 of 12 times cultured. This seemed to indicate that it was the blender that contaminated both milkshakes and feeding formulas. At that

TABLE 1. *Isolation of* P. aeruginosa *from food samples*

Foods	Samples examined	Samples positive	Samples positive with counts indicated[a]		
			10^1	10^2	10^3
Vegetable salads	115	52	30	18	4
Milkshakes	10	6	4	1	1
Feeding formulas[b]	34	9	7	2	0

[a] Per gram of vegetable salads; per ml of milkshakes and feeding formulas.
[b] Feeding formulas include nasogastric feeds, renal feeds, and blenderized feeds.

time, however, milk in half-gallon cartons had not been cultured. On subsequent culturing of 60 half-gallon cartons, 4 were found to contain *P. aeruginosa* in counts of 1 to 10 colonies/ml. Therefore, it would appear that the milk itself might also have contributed to the contamination of the milkshakes and feeding formulas.

VEGETABLES AS RESERVOIRS OF *P. AERUGINOSA*

Originally, we showed that *P. aeruginosa* was introduced into the salads served to patients through the vegetables used in preparation. The kitchen personnel did not introduce *P. aeruginosa* since cultures of hands were positive only when taken from personnel during handling of vegetables (6).

Elrod and Braun (3) reported that *P. aeruginosa* can cause disease in plants (sugar cane, tobacco, and lettuce) and Samish and Etinger-Tulczynska (11) reported on pseudomonads as normal flora of vegetables; thus, it was implied that *P. aeruginosa* is a saprophytic organism found in plants and foliage. Which of the vegetables, however, was the major source of the organism? An examination of vegetables received at the hospital was undertaken, with the supposition that, if only one or two vegetables were predominantly carrying *P. aeruginosa,* these could easily be eliminated from the patients' diet.

In this series of experiments, 85 vegetable samples obtained from the hospital's kitchen were cultured. These were in addition to 77 samples cultured originally (6). As shown in Table 2, *P. aeruginosa* was isolated from almost 30% of the samples. Tomatoes, celery, endive, and cucumbers showed the highest frequencies of recovery and the highest counts/g. Two samples (14%) from tomatoes yielded about 10^3 *Pseudomonas*/g. Also, 10^2 *Pseudomonas*/g were present in at least one sample each of celery, endive, cucumbers, radishes, and carrots, whereas all samples from cabbage and lettuce were negative for *P. aeruginosa*. Generally, there was a higher

TABLE 2. *Isolation of* P. aeruginosa *from vegetables*

Vegetable	Samples examined	Samples positive	Samples positive with indicated counts[a]		
			10^1	10^2	10^3
Tomato	16	5	3	0	2
Radish	8	1	0	1	0
Celery	17	9	5	4	0
Carrot	11	1	0	1	0
Endive	6	5	3	2	0
Cabbage	5	0	0	0	0
Cucumber	11	4	3	1	0
Lettuce	11	0	0	0	0

[a] Per gram of vegetable.

frequency of *P. aeruginosa* recovery in the previous study. However, such a difference could be caused by seasonal variations or by different geographical origins of the produce. No efforts were made to examine seasonal or geographical effects on the frequency of *P. aeruginosa* in vegetables.

The pyocin types of *P. aeruginosa* from vegetables are shown in Table 3. The most common types were D-2, B-7, F-2, and F-6. Pyocin typing of the isolates from specimens received at the clinical laboratory from patients throughout the hospital during the period of this study (Table 4) revealed many of the types to be identical to those recovered from vegetables. One type, B-6, however, was not recovered from vegetables in this series of experiments, although it was quite common among clinical isolates and it was a common isolate among vegetables cultured during our original studies (6).

In addition to *P. aeruginosa,* we isolated *Klebsiella, Enterobacter, Serratia,* and *Citrobacter* species from

TABLE 3. *Pyocin types of* P. aeruginosa
recovered from vegetables

Vegetable	No. isolates typed	Pyocin types							
		B-7	D-2	F-2	F-4	F-6	P-1	VT[a]	NT[b]
Tomato	78	9	39	6	2	6	2	12	2
Radish	3	—	—	—	—	—	—	3	—
Celery	29	5	9	—	—	—	5	10	—
Carrot	6	—	—	6	—	—	—	—	—
Endive	21	—	6	—	—	5	—	9	1
Cucumber	9	—	3	—	—	1	1	2	2
Total	146	14	57	12	2	12	8	36	5

[a] VT, variable type: unstable typing pattern.
[b] NT, nontypable: no inhibition of indicator strains.

TABLE 4. *Pyocin types of* P. aeruginosa *recovered from specimens of patients throughout the hospital*

Specimen	No. isolates typed	Pyocin types								
		B-6	B-7	D-2	F-2	F-4	F-6	P-1	VT[a]	NT[b]
Urine	118	6	21	32	16	3	10	2	19	9
Sputum	83	2	10	23	7	1	8	1	21	10
Wound	76	6	9	18	14	4	5	—	20	—
Blood	7	—	—	3	2	—	—	—	1	1
Total	284	14	40	76	39	8	23	3	61	20

[a] VT, variable type: unstable typing pattern.
[b] NT, nontypable: no inhibition of indicator strains.

vegetables. *Klebsiella* was recovered from more than 50% of vegetable samples with maximum counts of $10^4/g$ from tomatoes, radishes, celery, and cucumbers *(unpublished data)*. Since *E. coli* has not been recovered from any vegetables (or vegetable salads) examined thus far, we can eliminate fecal contamination as a means of introducing the bacteria to these products.

CONTROL OF *PSEUDOMONAS* INFECTIONS IN BURN PATIENTS VIA CONTROL OF DIET

In September 1973, we introduced a controlled diet for burn patients in which all food including fresh vegetables had to be cooked. Milkshakes were to be prepared in blenders that were previously washed in automatic dishwashers (190°F). Arrangements were made with a local dairy to provide the kitchen with milk pasteurized by flash heating at 300°F. (This milk was shown to be free of gram-negative bacteria.) After the controlled diet had been in use for over 1 year and with 80 patients treated in the burn center, as shown in Table 5, we had only 5 patients with *Pseudomonas* sepsis (6.25%). This is a significant reduction from the 32% rate of infection prior to the controlled diet ($p < 0.005$).

While the controlled diet was in effect, we noticed that feeding formulas prepared in the kitchen were contaminated with *P. aeruginosa, Klebsiella,* and *Enterobacter* (feeding formulas are also known as nasogastric, renal, or blenderized feeds). Table 1 shows the frequency of *P. aeruginosa* in the formulas examined (26%). Only one patient in the burn center had used nasogastric feeds that proved to be contaminated in retrospect. (The patient died from bronchial pneumonia shortly afterward.) There were, however, several other patients in different wards using these contaminated feeds. We immediately stopped the preparation of the feeding formulas in the kitchen and acquired commercially available products that were suitable for use.

PSEUDOMONAS AERUGINOSA INGESTION, COLONIZATION, AND INFECTION: A HYPOTHESIS

One important factor we considered in linking consumption of foods to *Pseudomonas* colonization and infection was the size of the inoculum. Was the inoculum via food consumption adequate to lead to colonization of the gastrointestinal tract? Vegetable salads harboring *P. aeruginosa* carry from 10^1 to 10^3 *Pseudomonas*/g. Therefore, a patient who consumes 80 g of salad (average portion) may ingest from 8×10^2 to 8×10^4 *Pseudomonas*. Shooter (13) has suggested that individuals consuming 10^4 or more *Pseudomonas* may become transitory carriers. Buck and Cooke (2) demonstrated that antibiotic treatment (ampicillin) in normal individuals prolonged

TABLE 5. *Effect of diet on* P. aeruginosa
infection in patients with burns

Patients	General diet[a]	Controlled diet[b]
Total no.	120	80
Infected with		
P. aeruginosa	38 (32%)	5 (6.25%)
Not infected with		
P. aeruginosa	82	75

[a] General diet was used from 8/71 to 9/73.
[b] Controlled diet was used from 10/73 to 3/75.

fecal carriage of ingested *P. aeruginosa,* whereas in people not taking antibiotics, excretion of this organism in feces was transient and never lasted beyond 48 to 72 hr after ingestion, even if 10^6 or more organisms were given. Most patients admitted to our burn center receive penicillin and streptomycin on admission and, in addition, during the hospital stay, they receive broad-spectrum antibiotics such as cephalothin, ampicillin, and kanamycin; as a result, they could be predisposed to gastrointestinal colonization with *P. aeruginosa.*

The mechanism by which antibiotics aid in colonization was explained by Levison (7) who showed that the gastrointestinal tract of mice is resistant to colonization due to short-chain fatty acids produced by the colon flora that are highly inhibitory to *P. aeruginosa.* Therefore, extensive use of antibiotics in patients could suppress the colon flora and, consequently, reduce or eliminate short-chain fatty acid production that would allow *Pseudomonas* colonization.

A hypothesis is proposed in which a cycle of events can be described for a mode of acquisition, infection, and transmission of *P. aeruginosa* in patients with burns. A patient may acquire *P. aeruginosa* from vegetable salads or contaminated diets. Aided by extensive antibiotic use, the organism may colonize the gastrointestinal tract. Autoinfection or endogenous infection may then take place and, if several patients are on the same diet, more than one patient would develop *Pseudomonas* infection. This sporadic outbreak can lead to a hyperendemic situation if hand washing is not enforced and instruments and equipment are not adequately sterilized. If all environmental factors and diets are controlled, the rate of infection would be very low (6%), as the only sources of *P. aeruginosa* are the few patients who were already colonized when admitted.

SUMMARY

In conclusion, there is ample evidence that *P. aeruginosa* is found in certain foods served to patients, and we have presented data that suggest that elimination or control of such foods served to patients with burns reduces *Pseudomonas* infection significantly. It would be of interest if other institutions with susceptible populations, such as patients with burns, leukemias, kidney transplants, etc., would introduce controlled diets to determine their effect on the incidence of *Pseudomonas* infection.

ACKNOWLEDGMENTS

We thank Ann Hunt and the dietary personnel of Mercy Hospital for their invaluable assistance in obtaining food samples.

We also appreciate the excellent technical assistance offered by Barbara Grosiak Rotz and Charles Wright.

REFERENCES

1. Alexander, J. W. (1971): Pseudomonas infections in man. In: *Proceedings of the International Conference on Nosocomial Infection.* American Hospital Association, Chicago, pp. 103–111.
2. Buck, A. C., and Cooke, E. M. (1969): The fate of ingested *Pseudomonas aeruginosa* in normal persons. *J. Med. Microbiol.*, 2:521–525.
3. Elrod, R. P., and Braun, A. C. (1942): *Pseudomonas aeruginosa; its role as a plant pathogen. J. Bacteriol.*, 44:633–644.
4. Kantor, L. T., Kominos, S. D., and Yee, R. B. (1975): Identification of nonfermentative gram-negative bacteria in the clinical laboratory. *Am. J. Med. Technol.*, 41:3–9.
5. Kominos, S. D., Copeland, C. E., and Grosiak, B. (1972): Mode of transmission of *Pseudomonas aeruginosa* in a burn unit and an intensive care unit in a general hospital. *Appl. Microbiol.*, 23:309.
6. Kominos, S. D., Copeland, C. E., Grosiak, B., and Postic, B. (1972): Introduction of *Pseudomonas aeruginosa* into a hospital via vegetables. *Appl. Microbiol.*, 24:567–570.
7. Levison, M. E. (1973): Effect of colon flora and short chain fatty acids on growth *in vitro* of *Pseudomonas aeruginosa* and *Enterobacteriaceae. Infect. Immun.*, 8:30–35.
8. Lowbury, E. J. L., and Fox, J. (1954): The epidemiology of infection with *Pseudomonas pyocyanae* in a burns unit. *J. Hyg.*, 52:403–416.
9. Lowbury, E. J. L., Thom, B. T., Lilly, H. A., Babb, J. R., and Whittall, K. (1970): Sources of infection with *Pseudomonas aeruginosa* in patients with tracheostomy. *J. Med. Microbiol.*, 3:39–56.
10. Parker, M. T. (1971): Causes and prevention of sepsis due to gram-negative bacteria: Ecology of the infecting organism. *Proc. Roy. Soc. Med.*, 64:979–980.
11. Samish, Z., and Etinger-Tulczynska, R. (1963): Distribution of bacteria within the tissue of healthy tomatoes. *Appl. Microbiol.*, 11:7–100.
12. Schimpff, S. C., Young, V. M., Greene, W. H., Vermeullen, G. D., Moody, M. R., and Weirnik, P. H. (1972): Origin of infection in acute nonlymphocytic leukemia. *Ann. Intern. Med.*, 77:707–714.
13. Shooter, R. H. (1971): Bowel colonization of hospital patients by *Pseudomonas aeruginosa* and *Escherichia coli. Proc. Roy. Soc. Med.*, 64:989–990.
14. Shooter, R. A., Cooke, E. M., Gaya, H., Kumar, P., Patel, N.,

Parker, M. T., Thom, B. T., and France, D. R. (1969): Food and medicaments as possible sources of hospital strains of *Pseudomonas aeruginosa. Lancet,* 1:1227–1229.

15. Shooter, R. A., Faiers, M. C., Cooke, E. M., Breaden, A. L., and O'Farrell, S. M. (1971): Isolation of *Escherichia coli, Pseudomonas aeruginosa,* and *Klebsiella* from foods in hospitals, canteens, and schools. *Lancet,* 2:390–393.

16. Shooter, R. A., Walker, K. A., Williams, V. R., Horgan, G. M., Parker, M. T., Asheshov, E. H., and Bullimore, J. F. (1966): Fecal carriage of *Pseudomonas aeruginosa* in hospitalized patients. *Lancet,* 2:1331–1334.

17. Smith, R. F., and Dayton, S. L. (1972): Use of acetamide broth in the isolation of *Pseudomonas aeruginosa* from rectal swabs. *Appl. Microbiol.,* 24:143–145.

18. Stoodley, B. J., and Thom, B. T. (1970): Observations on the intestinal carriage of *Pseudomonas aeruginosa. J. Med. Microbiol.,* 3:367–375.

19. Zabransky, R. J., and Day, F. E. (1969): Pyocine typing of clinical strains of *Pseudomonas aeruginosa. Appl. Microbiol.,* 17:293–296.

Pseudomonas aeruginosa: Ecological Aspects and Patient Colonization, edited by Viola Mae Young. Raven Press, New York © 1977.

Epidemiology of *Pseudomonas aeruginosa* in a Burns Hospital

Ian Alan Holder

Shriner's Burns Institute, and Departments of Microbiology and Surgery, University of Cincinnati College of Medicine, Cincinnati, Ohio 45219

In recent years, *Pseudomonas aeruginosa* infections have been incriminated as a major threat to compromised hosts in general and to burned patients in particular (10, 15,18,19). Some of the characteristics of this organism that have contributed to the potential danger of its infecting patients, or even being present in the environment where compromised patients are housed, are as follows: the organism has nonexacting nutritional requirements, is able to metabolize a variety of carbon sources, can utilize ammonium compounds as a nitrogen source, can multiply over a wide temperature range (10 to 43°C), is resistant to several widely used disinfectants and preservatives, and, finally, is resistant to a wide range of antibiotics.

EXOGENOUS SPREAD OF *P. AERUGINOSA*

Table 1 indicates that between 5 to 29% of the several hospitalized populations tested for fecal carriage were

TABLE 1.   Pseudomonas aeruginosa: *Carriage rates*

Source and percent of carriages		Population tested	Reference
Fecal	24%	Hospital patients on admission	Shooter et al. (13)
Fecal	29%	Pediatric patients	Henderson et al. (7)
Fecal	19%	Hospital patients 1st day on ward	Shooter et al. (14)
Fecal	5%	Burned patients on admission	Kefalides et al. (8)
Saliva	6.6%	Normal individuals	Sutter et al. (17)
Saliva	5%	Hospitalized patients	Shooter et al. (14)

positive for *P. aeruginosa*. The salivary carriage rate is approximately the same in hospitalized patients as it is in normal individuals. From these data, one may erroneously conclude that hospital-acquired infections from *P. aeruginosa* are probably endogenous in origin. However, this does not seem to be the case because it has been shown that in patients tested for *Pseudomonas* carriage 2 days post-admission to the hospital, 24% of the stool cultures were positive, but 38% of the stools of the patients in the study became positive at some time during the hospital stay (13). This indicates that 14% of the population in addition to the initial fecal carriers were colonized during their hospitalization and that this colonization was of exogenous origin.

More dramatic demonstration of the exogenous spread of *P. aeruginosa* infection in the hospital environment occurs when the population consists of patients who are highly susceptible to infection with *P. aeruginosa,* such as burned patients. A study involving burned patients similar to the one described above revealed that although only approximately 5% were fecal carriers of *Pseudomonas* on or shortly after admission, this percentage had risen to 20% on the fifth post-burn day, and by the twelfth post-burn day had reached 40% (8). More importantly, perhaps, skin colonization with *P. aeruginosa,* which on admission was between 5 to 10%, reached 65% by the third post-burn day and over 80% by the ninth post-burn day. These studies lend experimental support to the strong admonition of Sutter and Hurst (16) to those involved in the epidemiology of *Pseudomonas,* especially those concerned with burned patients: "Establishing patients, hospital environment and contacts as primary sources of infection in burns is an important step in prevention. As long as infections by pseudomonas are thought to arise from indigenous flora, disease caused by these bacteria will be considered inevitable in patients with extensive burns. When it is recognized that these infections are of exogenous origin and preventive measures taken, disease rates can be decreased."

Many potential sources of *P. aeruginosa* infection in the hospital environment have been reported. Table 2 gives a sample, by no means complete, of some that have been reported in the literature. Close examination of these studies reveals that the most common denominator in exogenous environmental sources of *P. aeruginosa* in hospitals is a moist environment.

Much of the methodology of environmental and epidemiological studies performed at the Shriner's Burns Institute, Cincinnati, Ohio, has been published previously (5,6) but is briefly summarized here.

TABLE 2. *Some reported sources of* P. aeruginosa *in the hospital environment*

Source	Reference
Bottled fluids	Lowbury, E. J. L. (9)
Disinfectants	Plotkin, S. A., and Austrian, R. (12)
	Burdon, D. W., and Whitby, J.L. (4)
Liquid soaps, antiseptic creams	Ayliffe et al. (1,2)
Baths and sinks	Henderson et al. (7)
Water faucets	Shooter et al. (14)
Resuscitation equipment	Basset et al. (3)

Serological Typing

Rabbit antiserum to each of the seven Parke-Davis immunotypes were used. A drop of antiserum was added to a saline suspension of the test culture on a microscope slide and observed for agglutination.

Bacteriophage Typing

Twenty-two phages and their homologous propagating strains were kindly supplied by M. T. Parker (Cross Infection Reference Laboratory, Central Public Health Laboratory, Colindale, N.W. 9, London, England). Lyophilized phages were reconstituted with Trypticase Soy Broth (TSB) and propagated in their homologous host strains. The routine test dilution (RTD) for each phage strain was determined on its respective host. Each test culture was grown in TSB for 2 hr at 32°C and inoculated onto the surface of a Trypticase Soy Agar plate (containing 1% purified agar) for confluent growth. Open plates were dried at room temperature for 1 hr. Then one drop of each phage RTD was added to each test culture. After phages had absorbed to the medium, plates were incubated at 32°C for 12 to 14 hr. The lytic patterns were scored as follows: confluent lysis, +++; 50 to 100 plaques, ++; 20 to 50 plaques, +; fewer than 20 plaques, ±. Only +++ and ++ scores were recorded as type reactions.

RECOVERY OF *P. AERUGINOSA*

Results of patients' cultures during the 3-month survey of these studies revealed that, of the 31 patients admitted to the hospital, 16 had cultures positive for *P. aeruginosa* while hospitalized (Fig. 1). Four of these 16 were positive when the study began, 3 others were positive on admission, and 9 developed *P. aeruginosa* during their hospital stay. These data reemphasize the exogenous aspect of the spread of *Pseudomonas* in the hospital environment.

DISTRIBUTION OF SEROTYPES

Figure 2 shows the distribution of serotypes in these patients for the same 3-month period. While types 1, 2, and 5 were the most prevalent types, they appeared to be randomly distributed among the patients. Patients D. R. and S. C. had populations of *P. aeruginosa* that were of different strains by serotyping, yet both patients were housed in close proximity to each other for a long period of time during which they were highly infected. Representative wound, urine, and body surface cultures consistently revealed that the *P. aeruginosa* isolated from each patient remained individually monospecific by

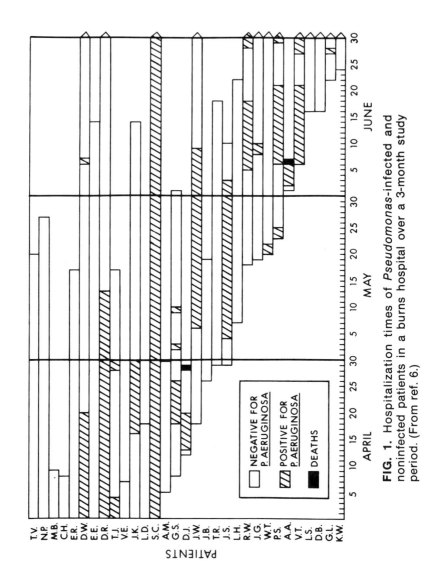

FIG. 1. Hospitalization times of *Pseudomonas*-infected and noninfected patients in a burns hospital over a 3-month study period. (From ref. 6.)

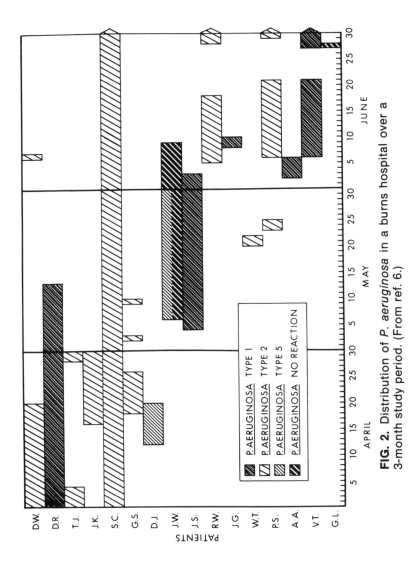

FIG. 2. Distribution of *P. aeruginosa* in a burns hospital over a 3-month study period. (From ref. 6.)

serotyping and distinctly different from each other by phage typing. Cross-contamination between patients was ruled out as a major source of spread of *Pseudomonas* as a consequence of these data.

ENVIRONMENTAL SOURCES OF *P. AERUGINOSA*

Since cross-contamination between patients had been ruled out, a search for other potential sources of *Pseudomonas* dissemination was initiated. It can be seen from Table 3 that several of the environmental sources tested were either totally negative or only occasionally positive for *P. aeruginosa*. Sink basins and particularly sink drains were frequently and consistently positive, as were drains from the whirlpool. Thirty-three to 48% of the cultures that were isolated from sinks were nontypable by serological methods. However, among those that were typable, serotypes 1 and 2 (the most common serotypes colonizing patients), were also the ones most commonly encountered in the sinks.

Although sinks appeared to be a major source of environmental *P. aeruginosa,* the link between this potential reservoir of infection and the patients could not be established from this study. The obvious vectors, nursing personnel, were not incriminated because cultures from their nasopharynx, hair, and hands in particular (see Table 3), were consistently negative. Therefore, additional studies were initiated in order to try to determine the vectors between the patients and the sinks. Table 4 shows the results of these studies. Again, the sinks appear to be a major reservoir for *Pseudomonas*. In this survey, as opposed to the previous study, a small number

TABLE 3. *Environmental sources of* P. aeruginosa *during a 3-month survey in 1971*[a]

Source	April	May	June
Air	0/8	0/8	0/8
Nebulizer H_2O	1/8	0/8	0/2
Counter surface	0/24	3/24	0/24
Bed rails	1/16	2/16	5/16
Nurses' hands	0/24	0/24	0/24
Sinks			
Drain	51/56	54/56	55/56
Basin	15/56	18/56	15/56
Faucet	0/56	0/56	0/56
Whirlpool			
Drain	7/12	9/16	4/12
Inside	2/12	1/16	0/16

[a] Expressed as the ratio of positive cultures per total cultures. (From Edmonds et al., ref. 6.)

TABLE 4. *Environmental cultures: Follow-up study*

Area cultured	No. of cultures	No. positive for *Pseudomonas*
Air samples	24	0
Nurses' hands	24	2
Sink basin	168	44
Sink trap	168	160
Sink faucet	160	1

of the cultures from nurses' hands were positive. It is interesting to note that the hand impression plates from the nurses who were positive for *P. aeruginosa* showed that the organisms were on the thumb and first finger, the two fingers that were used to turn the sink faucet on and off. The serotypes isolated were the same serotypes that were found on the faucets and in the sinks and were similar to types colonizing patients. It was also determined that the personnel whose hands yielded positive cultures of *Pseudomonas* sp. had been asked to make a hand impression on plates immediately after washing their hands. It was subsequently found that hands became culturally negative shortly after the moisture left after washing and drying had evaporated. This is important for those involved in the epidemiology of *Pseudomonas* to understand, because identification of the vector between environmental sources of the organism and the patient may not be found if the cultures are taken at the wrong time.

MODE OF SPREAD OF *P. AERUGINOSA*

These studies suggest that the *Pseudomonas* cycle in our hospital is as represented in Fig. 3. Ward personnel may pick up *Pseudomonas* from a moist environment, in our situation sinks, and then transfer organisms to the patient; alternatively, the ward personnel may carry the organisms from the patient to the moist environment (sink) and deposit them there in the process of washing hands. This completes the cycle and allows it to be perpetuated by other ward personnel. An additional way in which the cycle can be initiated, although less likely, is for the moist environment to be initially contaminated by the patient himself and, subsequently, ward personnel complete the cycle.

In a corollary study, it was shown that the splash from running water into a contaminated sink could be disseminated into the environment surrounding the sink. Figure 4 shows the results of one such experiment. It can be seen that *Pseudomonas*, which were contaminating the

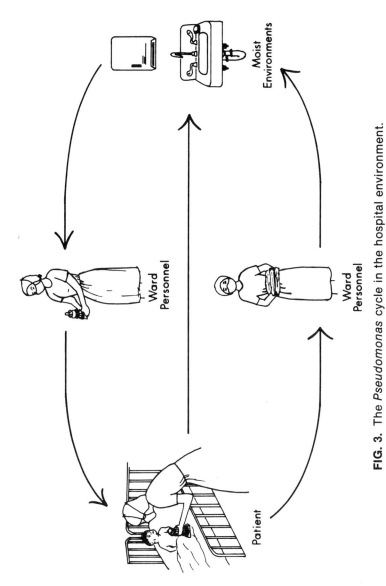

FIG. 3. The *Pseudomonas* cycle in the hospital environment.

Ward Personnel

Moist Environments

Ward Personnel

Patient

87

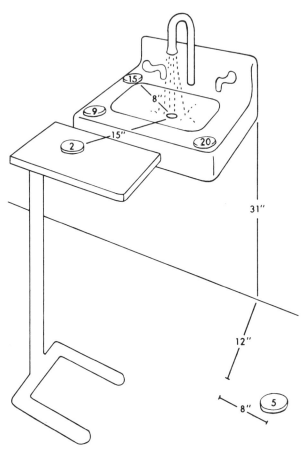

FIG. 4 Distribution pattern of *P. aeruginosa* caused by splash effect of running water in contaminated ward sink. The numbers on each of the plates represent the numbers of *Pseudomonas* collected during a 5-min splash study.

sink drain and basin, were transported into the environment by water droplets in fairly large numbers. Splash patterns obtained in this study indicated that water droplets could be splashed as far as 48 inches from the sink and, therefore, could potentially contaminate anything within that area.

CONTROL PROCEDURE

The following procedures were initiated to prevent the sinks from being a source of spread of *P. aeruginosa* and to break the *Pseudomonas* cycle. Aerators were installed on each sink and the flow of water was regulated to less than 6 liters/min to reduce splash. The aerator is removed at least once a month and soaked for 30 min in a 4%-acetic acid solution, rinsed, and then placed in 10% formalin for 10 min before being reused. This technique has been effective in maintaining pathogen-free aerators. The sink basins are cleaned at least once daily; twice-daily cleansing is done in areas where the infection potential is greatest, such as the intensive care unit. The basins are scrubbed with an abrasive cleaner and thoroughly rinsed. This is followed by the liberal application of a class-two disinfectant. Two-percent Vesphene was very useful in reduction of organisms to levels where dissemination no longer occurs. The disinfectant should be allowed to air dry before the sink is used to ensure maximum effective-

TABLE 5. *Dissemination of organisms from sinks before and after initiation of rigid cleansing procedures.*[a]

Method	Sink	*Pseudomonas* colonies developed	No. of plates
Not cleaned	W-4	11	4
	W-5	14	7
Cleaned	W-3	0	3
	W-1	0	7

[a] Samples taken at random.

TABLE 6. Sources of environmental contamination and control measures[a]

Source	Potential pathogens isolated	Dissemination	Control measure	Frequency
Patient	S. aureus Coliforms Yeast Other gram-negative rods P. aeruginosa Beta-hemolytic streptococcus	Contact: hands, body surface, wound Droplet: respiratory tract, urinary tract Particulate: hair, body surface	Appropriate antibiotics Necessary isolation	As required
Personnel	S. aureus Yeast Coliforms P. aeruginosa Other gram-negative rods	Contact: hands Droplet: respiratory tract Particulate: hair, body surface	Gowning change Hands: adequate washing, gloves Hair: washing with appropriate agent, covering Nares: mask, topical antibiotics	As required between patients
Sinks	Alcaligenes P. aeruginosa Gram-negative rods S. aureus	Droplet (splash): basin Harborage: aerator	Keep sinks dry: stop drips and leaks Regulate flow to 6 liters/minute Use aerators Clean sinks and aerators	Sinks: clean 1–2 times/day Aerators: change 1–2 times/month

90

Floors (specific areas)	S. aureus Yeast P. aeruginosa Gram-negative rods	Droplet nuclei: spills Particulate: dust	Frequent cleaning in high-risk areas Immediate clean-up of spills, especially contaminated material	Clean 2–3 times/day
Diet	Coliforms Other gram-negative rods P. aeruginosa Pseudomonas species	Ingestion Contact	Proper cooking Thorough wash Cold or dry storage	As required
Drugs, soaps, cosmetic items	Gram-negative rods P. aeruginosa	Ingestion Injection Contact	Do not use until cultured Remove suspect items Dispose of contaminated items	Spot checks As required On request
Blanketrol	Gram-negative rods P. aeruginosa	Contact: leaks, punctures	40% propylene glycol 100–250 ppm formalin	Fluid used in tank
Nebulizers and oxygen equipment	Gram-negative rods	Contact Inhalation	Sterilization Short-term usage	Between patients or as required
Hydrotherapy equipment	Gram-negative rods P. aeruginosa S. aureus	Contact: water, tub	Plastic liners Arm-length gloves Good housekeeping	As required
Air	Yeast P. aeruginosa S. aureus	Droplet nuclei Particulate	Maintain filters Single air pass Keep ducts and grates clean	Change yearly or when necessary As required

[a] In order of decreasing frequency.

91

ness. Dripping faucets are immediately repaired to reduce the moisture level on the basin surface. Data from
studies similar to the one outlined in Fig. 4 performed on
sinks before and after the above procedures were initiated are presented in Table 5. In the sinks treated by
the cleaning methods outlined, no *Pseudomonas* colonies
were isolated, whereas those tested before the cleaning
procedures were introduced showed a fair number of
Pseudomonas colonies developing on the test plates.

It should be obvious to the reader that patients, ward
personnel, and sinks are not the only links in the chain of
the *Pseudomonas* cycle in a burns hospital, nor is
Pseudomonas the only organism whose epidemiology is
important to understand in a burns hospital. Table 6
shows several potential sources of environmental contamination (in order of decreasing frequency), some of
the organisms isolated, and the control measure(s) used
to control their dissemination. Lowbury (11), in speaking
about cross-infection and acquired resistance in microorganisms, says " . . . indeed, within each species funda-
mental differences of behavior may be found and
generalizations . . . referring to all species are almost sure
to be wrong." I submit that generalizations about the
epidemiology of *Pseudomonas* from the studies cited
above would also be inappropriate, other than to be
aware and exercise surveillance (and, if necessary, control) of moist environments. The preceding descriptions
concern one situation that occurred in one burns hospital
and are presented to show some of the approaches that
were used to identify the epidemiological problems and
some of the methods used to resolve them. Table 6 is
presented to show potential sources of a variety of
nosocomial infections in our hospital and measures that

have been devised to control these infections. We believe that our procedures can serve as a guide for those involved in *Pseudomonas* surveillance and may be used for whatever specific needs arise in any particular institution.

SUMMARY

Data are presented from epidemiological studies on the mode of dissemination of *P. aeruginosa* in a burns unit. The results confirm other reports that the transmission of *Pseudomonas* in the hospital environment is of exogenous rather than endogenous nature. The cycle of *Pseudomonas* spread in the hospital environment appears to be from some moist environment, in our case sinks, that acts as a reservoir for the organisms to be transferred to the patients via ward personnel. The ward personnel then recontaminate the sink in the hand-washing process. Suggestions on how to interrupt this cycle are presented.

ACKNOWLEDGMENTS

Some of the data presented are from work done by Matthew Maley at the Shriner's Burns Institute and submitted to the Department of Civil and Environmental Engineering, University of Cincinnati, as part of the requirements for the Master of Science degree.

REFERENCES

1. Ayliffe, G. A. J., Lowbury, E. J. L., Hamilton, J. G., Small, J. M., Asheshov, E. A., and Parker, M. T. (1965): Hospital infection with *Pseudomonas aeruginosa* in neurosurgery. *Lancet*, 2:365–369.

2. Ayliffe, G. A. J., Brightwell, K. M., Collins, B., and Lowbury, E. J. L. (1969): Varieties of aseptic practice in hospital wards. *Lancet,* 2:1117–1120.
3. Basset, D. C. J., Thompson, S. A. S., and Page, B. (1965): Neonatal infections with *Pseudomonas aeruginosa* associated with contaminated resuscitation equipment. *Lancet,* 1:781–784.
4. Burdon, D. W., and Whitby, J. L. (1963): Contamination of hospital disinfectants with *Pseudomonas* species. *Br. Med. J.,* 2:153–155.
5. Edmonds, P., Suskind, R. R., MacMillan, B. G., and Holder, I. A. (1972): Epidemiology of *Pseudomonas aeruginosa* in a burns hospital: Evaluation of serological, bacteriophage and pyocin typing methods. *Appl. Microbiol.,* 24:213–218.
6. Edmonds, P., Suskind, R. R., MacMillan, B. G., and Holder, I. A. (1972): Epidemiology of *Pseudomonas aeruginosa* in a burns hospital: Surveillance by a combined typing system. *Appl. Microbiol.,* 24:219–225.
7. Henderson, A., MacLaurin, J., and Scott, J. M. (1969): Pseudomonas in a Glasgow baby unit. *Lancet,* 2:316–317.
8. Kefalides, N. A., Arana, J. A., Bajan, A., Velarde, N., and Rosenthal, S. M. (1964): Evaluation of antibiotic prophylaxis and gamma globulin, plasma, albumin, and saline-solution therapy in severe burns. *Ann. Surg.,* 159:496–506.
9. Lowbury, E. J. L. (1951): Contamination of cetrimide and other fluids with *Pseudomonas pyocyanea. Br. J. Industr. Med.,* 8:22–25.
10. Lowbury, E. J. L., and Fox, J. (1954): The epidemiology of infection with *Pseudomonas pyocyanea* in a burns unit. *J. Hyg.,* 52:403–416.
11. Lowbury, E. J. L. (1955): Cross-infection of wounds with antibiotic-resistant organisms. *Br. Med. J.,* 1:985–990.
12. Plotkin, S. A., and Austrian, R. (1958): Bacteremia caused by *Pseudomonas* sp. following the use of materials stored in solutions of a cationic surface active agent. *Am. J. Med. Sci.,* 235:621–627.
13. Shooter, R. A., Walker, K. A., Williams, V. R., Hogan, G. M., Parker, M. T., Ashesov, E. A., and Bullmore, J. F. (1966): Faecal carriage of *Pseudomonas aeruginosa* in hospital patients. *Lancet,* 2:1331–1334.
14. Shooter, R. A., Cooke, E. M., Gaya, H., Kumar, P., Patel, N., Parker, M. T., and France, D. R. (1969): Food and medicament as possible sources of hospital strains of *Pseudomonas aeruginosa. Lancet,* 1:1227–1229.

15. Shulman, J. A., Terry, P. M., and Hough, C. E. (1971): Colonization with gentamicin resistant *Pseudomonas aeruginosa* pyocine type 5 in a burn unit. *J. Infect. Dis.*, 124:518–523.
16. Sutter, V. L., and Hurst, V. (1965): Sources of *Pseudomonas aeruginosa* infection in burns. *Ann. Surg.*, 163:597–602.
17. Sutter, V. L., Hurst, V., and Landucci, A. O. J. (1966): *Pseudomonas* in human saliva. *J. Dent. Res.*, 45:1800–1805.
18. Tinne, J. E., Gordon, A. M., Bain, W. H., and Mackey, W. A. (1967): Cross-infection by *Pseudomonas aeruginosa* as a hazard of intensive surgery. *Br. Med. J.*, 4:313–315.
19. Yow, E. M. (1952): Development of *Proteus* and *Pseudomonas* infections during antibiotic therapy. *J.A.M.A.*, 149:1184–1188.

Pseudomonas aeruginosa: Ecological Aspects and Patient Colonization, edited by Viola Mae Young. Raven Press, New York © 1977.

Factors Influencing Colonization of the Gastrointestinal Tract with *Pseudomonas aeruginosa*

Matthew E. Levison

Division of Infectious Diseases; Allergy and Immunology, The Medical College of Pennsylvania, Philadelphia, Pennsylvania 19129

More than two decades ago, many articles described spontaneous bacteremia principally caused by *Pseudomonas aeruginosa* in total body-irradiated mice (26). In these mice, bacteremia occurs 1 week following irradiation at a time when the neutrophil count is lowest, but after the intestinal mucosal lesions are healed.

Studies demonstrated that these mice were infected orally with *Pseudomonas* from drinking water contaminated with these microorganisms. When 10^7 *Pseudomonas* were introduced into the gastrointestinal tracts of nonirradiated mice, *Pseudomonas* could not be detected in more than half of the animals and did not occur in numbers greater than 10^5 bacteria in either the upper or lower intestines by the third day after inoculation. Irradiated mice fed 10^7 *Pseudomonas* retained *Pseudomonas* in the intestine, and by the third day after gastrointestinal inoculation, the number of these organisms had actually increased in approximately one-third of the animals (15). These experiences in radiobiologic research with experimental animals are similar to clinical experiences.

It is clear that patients in the hospital often swallow food or drugs contaminated with *P. aeruginosa* (20,30). However, subsequent colonization of the intestinal tract rarely occurs in normal individuals (31,32). Buck and Cooke (6) found that very large numbers of *Pseudomonas* (10^6 or more) had to be ingested by healthy volunteers before these organisms could be demonstrated in feces. This dose of bacteria did not lead to colonization; the total number of *Pseudomonas* recovered in feces was a small proportion of the amount ingested and fecal excretion was transient. It is therefore apparent that there are potent host-defense mechanisms against colonization by *Pseudomonas* in the normal gastrointestinal tract. However, colonization has been reported to occur when an antibiotic was simultaneously administered to which *Pseudomonas* was resistant (6). If colonization does occur, invasive disease due to *Pseudomonas* becomes likely, especially in patients with granulocytopenia (29).

DEFENSE AGAINST COLONIZATION

Several mechanisms of defense against colonization of the gastrointestinal tract with exogenous bacteria have been demonstrated for intestinal pathogens, such as those that cause cholera, shigellosis, and salmonellosis. It is unknown whether most of these mechanisms are active in prevention of intestinal colonization with *Pseudomonas*.

In the fasting state in man, the stomach and upper small intestine normally contain very low numbers of microorganisms. The large intestine normally contains approximately 10^{11} bacteria per g, 99% of which are obligate anaerobes.

Gastric Acidity

Gastric acidity apparently plays a major role in decreasing contamination of the stomach and the small bowel by reducing the number of ingested bacteria that reach the small intestine. Oral inoculation of an enteric pathogen together with alkali to neutralize gastric acid is required to initiate experimental infection with relatively low inocula (25). In addition, *Salmonella* gastroenteritis is more likely to occur in patients with absent gastric acid (1). Such a gastric mechanism would probably interfere with colonization by *Pseudomonas,* although this has not been demonstrated clinically or experimentally (15).

Intestinal Motility

Rapid motility normally clears the small bowel of bacteria that survive exposure to gastric acidity. Experimental and clinical evidence has shown that bacterial overgrowth in the small bowel is usually associated with a delayed transit (7). Administration of drugs that slow intestinal motility is known to increase susceptibility to experimental infection with intestinal pathogens (25). In addition, clinical use of Lomotil® exacerbates symptoms of shigellosis (8). However, intestinal stasis was found not to be a factor in *P. aeruginosa* colonization of the intestinal tract of irradiated mice (15). Whether small bowel stasis enhances colonization by *Pseudomonas* in man is unknown.

Immunity

Immune mechanisms operating within the intestinal tract are potentially important in the ecology of normal intestinal microflora and in resistance to colonization by nonindigenous microorganisms, such as enteric pathogens.

Secretions elaborated by tissues contiguous with the external environment are particularly rich in immunoglobulin A (IgA). Secretory IgA is less sensitive to enzymatic degradation than is serum immunoglobulin, which would be of obvious advantage in gastrointestinal secretions (5). IgA in serum and secretions has antibody activity for a wide variety of substances. Secretory IgA may protect against the absorption of certain food antigens; for example, individuals deficient in IgA have a high frequency of circulating antibodies to milk proteins (33). Recent experiments in mice (14) indicate that IgA antibody against *Vibrio cholerae* interferes with the attachment of the organisms to the gastrointestinal mucosa and protects against experimental cholera. Such inhibition of adherence of IgA-coated bacteria also has been described for streptococci on oral epithelial cells (34) and for enteropathogenic *Escherichia coli* on intestinal mucosa (27). For an invasive pathogen that produces bacteremia such as *P. aeruginosa,* inhibition of adherence probably would impair its ability to penetrate the mucosa and render it more susceptible to intestinal mechanical clearing mechanisms. Whether this phenomenon is operative for *P. aeruginosa* is unknown.

Effect of Antibiotics and Bacterial Interference

It has been well documented that administration of antimicrobial agents increases susceptibility to experimental infection with enteric pathogens and also favors proliferation of *Pseudomonas* in the bowel of man. This suggests that the normal resident flora of the large bowel interferes with colonization by exogenous bacteria. Bohnhoff et al. (2) were able to produce *Salmonella* infection in mice that were pretreated with streptomycin. Similarly, Freter (10,11) found that mice and guinea pigs could be made susceptible to infection with *S. flexneri* and *V. cholerae* by oral administration of antibiotics which presumably eliminated components of the normal intestinal flora, permitting establishment of the pathogen. Subsequent introduction of an *E. coli* strain into the intestinal tract of the experimental animals resulted in elimination of the shigellae (11). Hentges and Freter (18) found that various bacteria, including *E. coli,* fed orally, suppressed the growth of *S. flexneri* in the intestine of mice pretreated with antibiotics. Formal et al. (9) reported similar findings in germfree guinea pigs that died after oral infection with *S. flexneri,* whereas animals contaminated with *E. coli* survived challenge with *Shigella.*

One of the possible mechanisms of bacterial interference at mucosal sites that normally have an indigenous microflora (such as the large intestine in man) is the close association of microorganisms of the normal flora with epithelial surfaces. This association may limit access of exogenous bacteria to the mucosa. For example, in mice, some microorganisms of the normal flora seem to colonize the mucin on the epithelial surfaces, whereas others apparently attach directly to epithelial cells (28). The associations seem quite stable. However, in mice given penicillin solution in place of drinking water, the lactobacilli normally layered on the nonsecreting keratinized epithelium of the stomach disappear, and yeast from the secreting epithelium colonizes the nonsecreting epithelium (28). When the penicillin treatment is discontinued, the lactobacilli displace the yeast from the nonsecreting epithelium. The displacement must occur by lactobacilli interfering either with multiplication of the yeast on the tissue or with attachment of the yeast cells to the keratin layer. The yeasts never populate the nonsecreting epithelium while lactobacilli are present. Such phenomena may also be involved in resistance to certain exogenous bacteria, as well as in regulation of the indigenous microbiota of the alimentary tract.

Bacterial interference may also result from depletion by the normal flora of an essential nutrient required by the pathogen, or the microflora may elaborate substances such as fatty acids or deconjugated bile salts that inhibit growth of the pathogen (13).

From *in vitro* experiments (12), Freter concluded that inhibition of *Shigella in vivo* was due to competition for a carbon source in the highly reduced environment of the mouse cecum. However, Hentges and co-workers (16,17,19) attributed the inhibition of *S. flexneri* to volatile short-chain fatty acids, produced by various components of the normal intestinal flora including *Bacteroides fragilis,* which interfere with *Shigella* multiplication at the pH levels and redox potential present in the culture medium. In studies of Maier et al. (23), the short chain fatty acid, acetic acid, inhibited metabolism of *Shigella*. The bacteria apparently were penetrated only by the undissociated form of the volatile fatty acid that predominates at lower pH levels.

The data of Bohnhoff et al. (3,4) and Meynell (24) indicate that volatile fatty acids, produced by the normal gut flora in mice (in particular, *Bacteroides*), interfere with multiplication of *Salmonella* in the intestine. Their experiments demonstrated that *Salmonella* multiplication was inhibited *in vitro* by suspensions of large intestinal contents from normal mice. Volatile fatty acids were recovered from the intestinal contents of the mice in concentrations that inhibited *Salmonella* growth *in vitro* at the pH level and redox potential of the intestines. Oral administration of streptomycin produced an increase in oxidation–reduction potential and pH of the intestinal contents accompanied by decrease in volatile fatty acid concentration and resulted in an increased susceptibility to *Salmonella* infection.

Volatile short-chain fatty acids may also regulate the normal flora. For example, when germ-free mice monocontaminated with *E. coli* were exposed to normal mice, anaerobic fusiform bacilli appeared in the large intestine of the formerly germ-free mice. This was correlated with the appearance of volatile fatty acids, especially butyric acid, in the intestinal contents, and with a 10^4-fold decline in numbers of *E. coli* (21). Penicillin feeding eliminated the anaerobic fusiforms from the large intestine. This was associated with the disappearance of significant levels of butyric acid and with a 10^6-fold increase in numbers of *E. coli,* suggesting that butyric acid produced by the anaerobic fusiform bacilli suppressed growth of *E. coli* in the large intestine.

RESISTANCE TO INTESTINAL COLONIZATION WITH *PSEUDOMONAS AERUGINOSA*

In a series of experiments in our laboratory, we investigated the role of the normal large bowel flora in the resistance of the intestine to colonization with a strain of *P. aeruginosa* isolated from the blood of a patient (22).

Effect of pH

Heat-stable antibacterial activity in the following suspensions was demonstrated against *P. aeruginosa* at pH 6.5, 6.0, and 5.5: (a) pooled colon contents of normal mice; (b) an anaerobic, 48-hr culture of normal mouse feces; and (c) 48-hr cultures of different bacteria from human colon flora *(E. coli, B. fragilis, Klebsiella pneumoniae,* and *Proteus mirabilis).* The inhibition was not caused by depletion of nutrients, as the filtrates were supplemented with fresh nutrient broth. The antibacterial activity was affected by pH; that is, the lower the pH the greater the antibacterial activity. Inhibition at the lower pH levels was not simply caused by the acidity of the medium, because broth controls buffered at pH 5.5 never inhibited multiplication of *P. aeruginosa.* This suggested that weak acids, such as the short-chain fatty acids which are produced by fecal microorganisms, were the antibacterial substances.

Fatty Acids

The antibacterial activity of five fatty acids (propionic, butyric, isobutyric, acetic, and formic acids) was greater against *P. aeruginosa* than against three *Enterobacteriaceae (E. coli, K. pneumoniae,* and *P. mirabilis)* at all fatty acid concentrations (0.16 M to 0.005 M) and at the three pH values studied (5.5, 6.0, and 6.5). As the pH value increased, the antibacterial activity decreased. Antibacterial activity was greater at higher fatty acid concentrations, and at each pH value it was greatest for the fatty acids having the highest pK_a values. Lactic acid, with the lowest pK_a, exhibited little or no antibacterial activity. The dependence of the inhibitory effect on the pK_a of the fatty acid and on the pH of the medium suggests that the undissociated acid molecule is the inhibitory agent. Table 1 shows the percentage of undissociated molecules for each of the fatty acids studied at the three pH values. The acids with the highest pK_a (propionic, isobutyric, butyric, and acetic acids) have the

TABLE 1. *Short-chain fatty acids, their pK_a, and percent of undissociated fraction at pH 6.5, 6.0, and 5.5*

Fatty acid	pK_a	Percent undissociated		
		pH 6.5	pH 6.0	pH 5.5
Propionic acid	4.87	2.3	6.9	18.9
Isobutyric acid	4.84	2.1	6.4	17.9
Butyric acid	4.81	2.0	6.0	16.9
Acetic acid	4.75	1.7	5.3	15.1
Formic acid	3.75	0.2	0.6	1.7
Lactic acid	3.08	0.04	0.1	0.4

greatest percentage of undissociated molecules at any pH value, and the percentage increases with decreasing pH. Among propionic, isobutyric, butyric, and acetic acids, there are only small differences in pK_a's and percent of undissociated molecules at each pH. Similarly, there were only small differences in antibacterial activity. Acetic and butyric acids, two of the three predominant volatile fatty acids determined by gas chromatography in the mouse colon contents and in the anaerobic culture of mouse feces, occurred *in vivo* in concentrations that inhibited growth of *P. aeruginosa in vitro* at the pH of the mouse cecum. These results suggest that undissociated short-chain fatty acids produced by the colon flora may be a mechanism of intestinal resistance to colonization by *P. aeruginosa*.

SUMMARY

In summary, several mechanisms that may prevent colonization of the gastrointestinal tract by potential pathogens have been reviewed. Evidence was presented that supports the concept that short-chain fatty acids in the undissociated state, produced by enteric bacteria, inhibit growth of *P. aeruginosa* and, to a lesser degree, certain members of the *Enterobacteriaceae*. This inhibitory effect may explain, in part, the resistance of the intestinal tract to colonization with *P. aeruginosa*. The other potential mechanisms of defense, such as secretory IgA, have not been demonstrated for *Pseudomonas*.

REFERENCES

1. Bennett, I. L., Jr., and Hook, E. W. (1959): Infectious diseases (some aspects of salmonellosis). *Ann. Rev. Med.,* 10:1–20.
2. Bohnhoff, M., Drake, B. L., and Miller, C. P. (1954): Effect of

streptomycin on susceptibility of intestinal tract to experimental salmonella infection. *Proc. Soc. Exp. Biol. Med.,* 86:132–137.

3. Bohnhoff, M., Miller, C. P., and Martin, W. R. (1964): Resistance of the mouse's intestinal tract to experimental salmonella infection. I. Factors which interfere with the initiation of infection by oral inoculation. *J. Exp. Med.,* 120:805–816.

4. Bohnhoff, M., Miller, C. P., and Martin, W. R. (1964): Resistance of the mouse's intestinal tract to experimental salmonella infection. II. Factors responsible for its loss following streptomycin treatment. *J. Exp. Med.,* 120:817–828.

5. Brown, W. R., Newcomb, R. W., and Ishizaka, K. (1970): Proteolytic degradation of exocrine and serum immunoglobulins. *J. Clin. Invest.,* 49:1374–1380.

6. Buck, A. C., and Cooke, E. M. (1969): The fate of ingested *Pseudomonas aeruginosa* in normal persons. *J. Med. Microbiol.,* 2:521–525.

7. Donaldson, R. M., Jr. (1970): Small bowel bacterial overgrowth. *Adv. Intern. Med.,* 16:191–212.

8. Dupont, H. L., and Hornick, R. B. (1973): Adverse effect of lomotil therapy in shigellosis. *J.A.M.A., 226:1525*–1528.

9. Formal, S. B., Dammin, G., Sprinz, H., Kundel, D., Schneider, H., Horowitz, R. E., and Forbes, M. (1961): Experimental shigella infections. V. Studies in germ-free guinea pigs. *J. Bacteriol.,* 82:284–287.

10. Freter, R. (1955): The fatal enteric cholera infection in the guinea pig, achieved by inhibition of normal enteric flora. *J. Infect. Dis.,* 97:57–65.

11. Freter, R. (1956): Experimental enteric Shigella and Vibrio infections in mice and guinea pigs. *J. Exp. Med.,* 104:411–418.

12. Freter, R. (1962): *In vivo* and *in vitro* antagonism of intestinal bacteria against *Shigella flexneri.* II. The inhibitory mechanism. *J. Infect. Dis.,* 110:38–46.

13. Freter, R., and Abrams, G. D. (1972): Function of various intestinal bacteria in converting germfree mice to the normal state. *Infect. Immun.,* 6:119–126.

14. Fubara, E. S., and Freter, R. (1973): Protection against enteric bacterial infection by secretory IgA antibodies. *J. Immunol.,* 111:395–403.

15. Hammond, C. W., Ruml, D., Cooper, D. B., and Miller, C. P. (1955): Studies on susceptibility to infection following ionizing radiation. III. Susceptibility of the intestinal tract to oral inoculation with *Pseudomonas aeruginosa. J. Exp. Med.,* 102:403–411.

16. Hentges, D. J. (1967): Inhibition of *Shigella flexneri* by the

normal intestinal flora. I. Mechanism of inhibition by Klebsiella. *J. Bacteriol.,* 93:1369–1373.

17. Hentges, D. J. (1969): Inhibition of *Shigella flexneri* by the normal intestinal flora. II. Mechanisms of inhibition by coliform organisms. *J. Bacteriol.,* 97:513–517.
18. Hentges, D. J., and Freter, R. (1962): *In vivo* and *in vitro* antagonism of intestinal bacteria against *Shigella flexneri.* I. Correlation between various tests. *J. Infect. Dis.,* 110:30–37.
19. Hentges, D. J., and Maier, B. R. (1970): Inhibition of *Shigella flexneri* by the normal intestinal flora. III. Interactions with *Bacteroides fragilis* strains *in vitro. Infect. Immun.,* 2:364–370.
20. Kominos, S. D., Copeland, C. E., Grosiak, B., and Postic, B. (1972): Introduction of *Pseudomonas aeruginosa* into a hospital via vegetables. *Appl. Microbiol.,* 24:567–570.
21. Lee, A., and Gemmell, E. (1972): Changes in the mouse intestinal microflora during weaning: Role of volatile fatty acids. *Infect. Immun.,* 5:1–7.
22. Levison, M. E. (1973): Effect of colon flora and short-chain fatty acids on growth *in vitro* of *Pseudomonas aeruginosa* and *Enterobacteriaceae. Infect. Immun.,* 8:30–35.
23. Maier, B. R., Onderdonk, A. B., Baskett, R. C., and Hentges, D. J. (1972): *Shigella,* indigenous flora interactions in mice. *Am. J. Clin. Nutr.,* 25:1433–1440.
24. Meynell, G. G. (1963): Antibacterial mechanisms of the mouse gut. II. The role of Eh and volatile fatty acids in the normal gut. *Br. J. Exp. Pathol.,* 44:209–219.
25. Miller, C. P., and Bohnhoff, M. (1962): A study of experimental *Salmonella* infection in the mouse. *J. Infect. Dis.,* 111:107–116.
26. Miller, C. P., Hammond, C. W., and Tompkins, M. (1951): The role of infection in radiation injury. *J. Lab. Clin. Med.,* 38:331–343.
27. Rutter, J. M., and Jones, G. W. (1973): Protection against enteric disease caused by *Escherichia coli*—a model for vaccination with a virulence determinant? *Nature (Lond.),* 242:531–532.
28. Savage, D. C. (1970): Associations of indigenous microorganisms with gastrointestinal mucosal epithelia. *Am. J. Clin. Nutr.,* 23:1495–1501.
29. Schimpff, S. C., Moody, M., and Young, V. M. (1970): Relationship of colonization with *Pseudomonas aeruginosa* to development of *Pseudomonas* bacteremia in cancer patients. *Antimicrob. Ag. Chemother.,* 10:240–244.
30. Shooter, R. A., Cooke, E. M., Faiers, M. C., Breaden, A. L., and

O'Farrell, S. M. (1971): Isolation of *Escherichia coli, Pseudomonas aeruginosa* and *Klebsiella* from food in hospitals, canteens and schools. *Lancet,* 2:390–392.

31. Shooter, R. A., Walker, K. A., Williams, V. R., Horgan, G. M., Parker, M. T., Asheshov, E. H., and Bullimore, J. F. (1969): Faecal carriage of *Pseudomonas aeruginosa* in hospital patients. *Lancet,* 2:1331–1334.

32. Stoodley, B. J., and Thom, B. T. (1970): Observations on the intestinal carriage of *Pseudomonas aeruginosa. J. Med. Microbiol.,* 3:367–375.

33. Tomasi, T. B., Jr., and Katz, L. (1971): Human antibodies against bovine immunoglobulin M in IgA deficient sera. *Clin. Exp. Immunol.,* 9:3–10.

34. Williams, R. C., and Gibbons, R. J. (1972): Inhibition of bacterial adherence by secretory immunoglobulin A: A mechanism of antigen disposal. *Science,* 177:697–699.

Pseudomonas aeruginosa: Ecological Aspects and Patient Colonization, edited by Viola Mae Young. Raven Press, New York © 1977.

Effect of Acquisition on the Incidence of *Pseudomonas aeruginosa* in Hospitalized Patients

Marcia R. Moody

Baltimore Cancer Research Center, National Cancer Institute, Baltimore, Maryland 21201

Acquisition of opportunistic pathogens by hospitalized patients has become a serious problem in the past decade. Infections caused by acquired bacteria have become frequent, especially in patients with severe underlying diseases (4). These infections are common and frequently cause death in patients with acute leukemias (10,18,19,20,21,24), renal transplants (1), burns (17), and severe traumas (22). Nosocomial infection has been shown to be associated with specific predisposing factors such as corticosteroids (8), broad-spectrum antibiotics (5,12,16), cancer chemotherapeutic or immunosuppressive agents (18,19,20), tracheostomies (11), contaminated water (13), respirators (14), and disinfectants (3). The many routes by which these organisms gain entrance to, and eventually become established in, the hospital environment have been discussed elsewhere in this monograph.

111

Schimpff et al. (20) have reported that 47% of the microbiologically documented infections in acute nonlymphocytic leukemia patients was caused by microorganisms that were acquired from the hospital environment and had become established as part of the patients' resident flora. It has also been noted that pharyngeal colonization with gram-negative bacilli was related to the severity of illness in certain hospitalized patients (9). Selden and co-workers (23) have shown that patients who acquired *Klebsiella* sp. after admission to a general hospital were prone to colonization of the intestinal tract by this organism, which led to a high incidence of later *Klebsiella* infections. Bacteremias were common in patients undergoing therapy in specialized cancer centers who acquired and became colonized with *Pseudomonas aeruginosa* (2,7,20). Thus, colonization of patients by these acquired strains appeared to have a direct bearing on infection.

As infection by *P. aeruginosa* is one of the major causes of morbidity and mortality in cancer patients (21), a rational design of measures that might reduce and/or prevent infections will depend largely on knowledge of the natural history of this microorganism. The patient population at the Baltimore Cancer Research Center (BCRC) consists of persons with leukemias, lymphomas, brain tumors, and metastatic solid tumors. Investigations on the incidence of *P. aeruginosa* in these patients (15,25) have been greatly facilitated in recent years by a rapid and reproducible serotying system developed by Fisher et al. (6). Serotyping has made it possible to evaluate the *P. aeruginosa* serotypes that were recovered from various groups of cancer patients in our hospital, to determine rates of acquisition of the serotypes by the patient groups, and to establish the effects of acquisition on the rate of colonization and/or subsequent infection in these patients.

METHODS FOR THE DETERMINATION OF ACQUISITION

In 1969 to 1970, admission and twice-weekly surveillance cultures of rectum, gingiva, axilla, nose, and urine from 190 cancer patients were evaluated as to their effectiveness in the epidemiological investigation of bacterial colonization and acquisition, and they were found to be generally sufficient to detect *P. aeruginosa* colonization and/or acquisition (18). These cultures, as well as diagnostic specimens taken when indicated, were useful in the separation of endogenous admission flora from acquired flora that had become part of the patient's resident flora. This method of taking two or more separate sets of cultures during the first 2 weeks of hospitalization greatly reduces the possibility of not detecting organisms that are present at admission. Conversely, the method probably lowers the actual acquisition rate of bacteria, as organisms acquired during the first few days in the hospital would be defined as present at admission. However, our experience has shown that extensive culturing to define admission flora yields results supporting the concept that microorganisms first detected after the initial 2 weeks of hospitalization are indeed acquired.

Admission and twice-weekly surveillance cultures were therefore used in this study to detect strains of *P. aeruginosa* that were part of the patients' admission flora and that were acquired during hospitalization. Bacteria that were recovered during the initial 2 weeks of the first hospital admission (two or more complete sets of cultures) were defined as "present at admission" or "not acquired," and those organisms that were detected for the first time after the initial 2 weeks of hospitalization were designated as "acquired." Colonization was defined as repeated recovery of a serotype from the same site, or different sites, on three or more separate occasions. Only documented infections were included in this report and were defined as having definite signs and symptoms of infection as well as cultural verification by the recovery of a causative organism from the blood or local site. The cultural data from these surveillance and diagnostic cultures form the basis of this report.

ACQUISITION RATES OF *P. AERUGINOSA*

Pseudomonas aeruginosa was recovered from 328 cancer patients at the BCRC during a 5-year study that ended in mid-1973 (Table 1). A total of 152 patients (46.3%) was found to be harboring this microorganism on admission. During subsequent hospitalizations, 47 of these patients (14.3%) also acquired another serotype of this organism, and 176 patients, from whom no *P. aeruginosa* was recovered at admission, also acquired strains of this bacterium during their hospital stay. In total, 68% of the cancer patients from whom *P. aeruginosa* was recovered acquired the strain after admission ($p < 0.001$). Moreover, patients in the leukemia–myeloma or solid tumor group were more likely to acquire *P. aeruginosa* than for it to be present in admission flora ($p < 0.001$ for both groups), whereas the recovery rate among lymphoma patients was not influenced by hospitalization.

TABLE 1. *Incidence of P. aeruginosa in 328 cancer patients*[a]

Diagnosis	Present at admission		Present at admission and acquired[c]		Acquired		Total no./ diagnosis
	No.	(%)[b]	No.	(%)	No.	(%)	
Leukemias and mye-lomas	38	(27.3)	19	(13.7)	82	(59.0)*[d]	139
Lymphomas	27	(36.0)	15	(20.0)	33	(44.0)	75
Solid Tumors	40	(35.1)	13	(11.4)	61	(53.5)*	114
Totals	105	(32.0)	47	(14.3)	176	(53.7)*	328

[a] Each patient counted once, that is, included in only one of the three categories shown on the table.
[b] Percentages based on total number per diagnosis.
[c] One serotype of *P. aeruginosa* was recovered from admission cultures and another serotype was recovered after the initial first 2 weeks of hospitalization.
[d] Kolmogorov-Smirnov one-sample test was used for statistical analysis. Asterisks denote *p* < 0.001.

From these cancer patients, 475 strains of *P. aeruginosa* were recovered (Table 2). Because of the higher acquisition recovery rates in these patients, it was not unexpected that the number of acquired strains (308; 64.8%), would be significantly higher than the number of strains present on admission (167; 35.2%). More than 59% of the strains recovered from each individual cancer patient group was acquired, and the acquisition frequencies of these strains were statistically higher among the leukemia–myeloma and solid tumor groups.

It was next determined whether a serotype would be more likely to be acquired by a specific patient group (Table 3). Recovery of a strain of *P. aeruginosa* serotype 5 or 7 from a patient in the leukemia–myeloma group would almost invariably indicate hospital acquisition, as 80% of the former serotype (p 0.0037) and 88.2% of the latter ($p < 0.0001$) were not present in admission flora of these patients. More strains of serotypes 1 and 4 were also acquired by these patients than were recovered from them at admission. Among solid tumor patients, serotypes 7 (p 0.0139), 6 (p 0.0244), and 1 (p 0.0287) were more likely to be acquired. Acquisition of serotype 2 by the lymphoma patient was quite common (80%, p 0.0287), an unusual finding as it was the serotype least often acquired by the other patient groups.

In most instances, the acquisition frequency of a particular serotype in one group did not differ appreciably from its frequency in the other patient groups. However, the leukemia–myeloma patient group acquired serotypes 1 and 7 more often than did the lymphoma patient group (p 0.027 and 0.028, respectively). In comparing the total strains acquired by the different groups, the leukemia, myeloma, or solid tumor patient acquired more strains of

TABLE 2. *Frequency of P. aeruginosa serotypes in a cancer population*[a]

Diagnosis	Present at admission		Acquired		Total no./diagnosis
	No.	(%)[b]	No.	(%)	
Leukemias and myelomas	61	(30.2)	141	(69.8)**c	202
Lymphomas	46	(40.7)	67	(59.3)	113
Solid tumors	60	(37.5)	100	(62.5)*	160
Totals	167	(35.2)	308	(64.8)**	475

[a] Each serotype per patient was counted once regardless of multiple recoveries of the particular serotype.
[b] Percentages based on total number per diagnosis.
[c] Kolmogorov-Smirnov one-sample test was used for statistical analysis. Asterisks denote the following *p* values: * < 0.025, ** < 0.001.

P. aeruginosa during hospitalization than did the lymphoma patient.

TRANSITORY STRAINS OF *P. AERUGINOSA*

It was of importance to establish whether certain strains of *P. aeruginosa* tended to be transitory and did not infect or colonize the cancer patient and whether acquisition affected this transiency, as such strains would be of little significance in the clinical management of the patient (Table 4).

An analysis of the data showed that, overall, acquisition did not appear to influence this tendency, as 38.3% of the strains recovered at admission and 31.9% of the acquired strains did not colonize or infect any patient, nor were there significant differences between the nonacquired and acquired frequencies of the various serotypes. However, this was not always the case in the individual cancer groups. Strains of serotype 4 that were present in admission cultures of the leukemia–myeloma patient group were usually transitory (71.4%), whereas only 13.3% of the acquired strains were transient (p 0.0136). The total strains that were recovered from lymphoma patients on entering the hospital were also more likely to be transitory in this group than were the total acquired strains (p 0.043).

When the question of transient serotypic behavior was considered, it became apparent that among the strains that were recovered from admission cultures, a serotype could demonstrate predilection for transiency, whereas among acquired strains, either the same or another serotype could also exhibit this behavior. But it is important to remember that in all groups, there were serotypes whose incidences appeared to be sufficiently high as to

TABLE 3. Serotypic acquisitions of P. aeruginosa by cancer patient groups

Serotype	Leukemias and myelomas			Lymphomas			Solid tumors		
	Total no. patients	Acquired No.	(%)	Total no. patients	Acquired No.	(%)	Total no. patients	Acquired No.	(%)
1	53	37	(69.8)***[a]	29	13	(44.8)	40	26	(65.0)*
2	31	17	(54.8)	10	8	(80.0)*	21	10	(47.6)
3	12	7	(58.3)	11	8	(72.7)	14	8	(57.1)
4	22	15	(68.2)*	8	6	(75.0)	20	12	(60.0)
5	20	16	(80.0)***	10	6	(60.0)	15	9	(60.0)
6	26	17	(65.4)	22	12	(54.5)	21	15	(71.4)*
7	34	30	(88.2)****	22	14	(63.6)	25	18	(72.0)*
Total	198	139	(70.2)	112	67	(59.8)	156	98	(62.8)

[a] A one-tailed Z-test was used to test difference between proportions for each serotype. Nontypable strains were not included. Asterisks denote the following p values: * $\leqq 0.05$, ** $\leqq 0.01$, *** < 0.005, **** < 0.001.

119

TABLE 4. *Frequencies of P. aeruginosa serotypes that did not colonize or infect patients in a cancer population*

Serotype	Leukemias–myelomas		Lymphomas		Solid tumors	
	Not acq.	Acq.	Not acq.	Acq.	Not acq.	Acq.
1	18.8[a]	24.3[a]	50.0	30.8	42.9	42.3
2	28.6	29.4	0.0	50.0	54.5	30.0
3	20.0	57.0	66.7	25.0	50.0	50.0
4	71.4[*b]	13.3	0.0	33.3	50.0	58.3
5	25.0	50.0	25.0	33.3	66.7	22.2
6	33.3	47.1	50.0	16.7	0.0	20.0
7	0.0	16.6	50.0	14.3	28.6	44.4
Total	28.8	29.5	44.4*	26.9	43.1	38.8

[a] Percentages based on the following: n/total no. nonacquired per serotype and n/total no. acquired per serotype.
[b] A two-tailed test was used to test differences between proportions. The asterisks denote the p value of < 0.05.

120

warrant comment (e.g., 57% for acquired serotype 3 in the leukemia−myeloma group, 66.7% for nonacquired serotype 3 in the lymphoma group); however, the percentages reflect too few patients to be statistically significant. Of these serotypes whose incidences were significant, strains of serotype 4 that were present at admission in the leukemia−myeloma group usually did not colonize or infect these patients (p 0.0078); conversely, acquired strains of serotypes 5 (p 0.017) and 6 (p 0.0255) were also more likely to be transitory than they were to colonize and/or infect this group. In general, admission strains among lymphoma patients were transient (p 0.0015), and specifically, so were the strains of serotype 1 (p 0.017). The nonacquired strain of *P. aeruginosa* as well as the acquired strain, in most instances, did not tend to infect or colonize the solid tumor patient (nonacquired, p 0.0008 and acquired, p 0.0006). It was also unlikely that serotype 1 (regardless of its acquisition status), nonacquired strains of serotypes 2 and 5, or acquired strains of serotypes 4 and 7 would infect or colonize these patients.

In comparing the total numbers of strains (nonacquired and acquired) that were transient in the patient groups, it was apparent that noncolonizing and/or noninfecting strains of *P. aeruginosa* were more prevalent in the solid tumor group (40.4%) than they were in the leukemia—myeloma group (29.3%, p 0.0193), whereas the incidence of these strains in the lymphoma patient (33.9%) did not differ significantly from those of the other groups.

COLONIZATION AND INFECTION BY *P. AERUGINOSA* IN THE CANCER PATIENT

In contrast to the solid tumor patients in whom most strains of *P. aeruginosa* were transitory and posed little threat of infection, the leukemia–myeloma group of cancer patients frequently became colonized with *P. aeruginosa* and infected with the same serotype (Table 5). The incidence of acquired strains that colonized and infected these patients (42.4%) was approximately the same as that of strains that were recovered on admission (44.8%). Similarly, no appreciable differences were noted in the frequencies of nonacquired and acquired strains that colonized these patients without infecting them or that infected them without prior colonization.

However, if *P. aeruginosa,* regardless of whether it was acquired or not, was recovered from these leukemia or myeloma patients, they usually became colonized and infected (nonacquired, p 0.0004 and acquired, p 0.00365), but rarely became colonized solely or infected without prior colonization. Acquired strains of serotype 1 had a decided tendency to colonize and infect these patients (51.3%, p 0.0002) and not to colonize them without causing infection (10.8%, p 0.0419). Nonacquired and acquired strains of serotype 7 invariably colonized and infected the leukemia–myeloma patient group. It would appear that this serotype has a high infectious potential, as 70% of the patients who acquired it became infected, irrespective of prior colonization (as did all four patients from whom it was recovered on admission).

Acquisition of a *P. aeruginosa* strain did not pose a greater threat of infection in lymphoma patients than did the nonacquired strain, as the incidence of strains acquired by lymphoma patients that colonized, colonized and infected, or infected them without colonization did not differ significantly from the corresponding incidence of nonacquired strains. As previously mentioned, nonacquired strains as well as acquired strains did demonstrate

TABLE 5. *Frequencies of P. aeruginosa serotypes that colonized and/or infected patients in a cancer population*

Sero-type	Leukemias–myelomas						Lymphomas						Solid tumors					
	Colonization only		Colonization and infection		Infection only		Colonization only		Colonization and infection		Infection only		Colonization only		Colonization and infection		Infection only	
	Not acq.[a]	Acq.[a]	Not acq.	Acq.	Not acq.	Acq.	Not acq.	Acq.	Not acq.	Acq.	Not acq.	Acq.	Not acq.	Acq.	Not acq.	Acq.	Not acq.	Acq.
1	31.3[b]	10.8**	37.5	51.3[c],****	12.5	13.5	25.0	23.1	6.3	0.0	18.8	46.2**	0.0	19.2	35.7	15.4	21.4	23.1
2	14.3	11.8	42.9	41.2	14.3	17.6	50.0	0.0	50.0	37.5	0.0	12.5	18.2	0.0	9.1	30.0	18.2	40.0
3	20.0	14.3	40.0	28.6	20.0	0.0	0.0	50.0	33.3	12.5	0.0	0.0	33.3	12.5	16.7	12.5	0.0	25.0
4	0.0	20.0	28.6	40.0	0.0	26.7	0.0	16.7	100.0	33.3	0.0	16.7	12.5	8.3	12.5	25.0	25.0	8.3
5	0.0	12.5	50.0	25.0	25.0	12.5	25.0	0.0	25.0	50.0	25.0	16.7	33.3	33.3	0.0	22.2	0.0	22.2
6	11.1	5.9	55.6	35.3	0.0	11.8	10.0	16.7	20.0	33.3	20.0	33.3	16.7	13.3	33.3	26.7	50.0	40.0
7	0.0	13.3	75.0*	50.0***	25.0	20.0	0.0	7.1	50.0	57.1*	0.0	21.4	42.9[a]	5.5	14.3	33.3	14.3	16.7
Totals	15.3	12.2	44.8****	42.4**	11.9	15.8	15.6	16.4	26.7	31.3	13.3	25.4	19.0	13.3	19.0	23.5	19.0	24.5

[a] A two-tailed test was used to compare differences between nonacquired and acquired strains. Serotype 7 that was present on admission was more likely to colonize the solid tumor patient than was the acquired strain of serotype 7 (p 0.022). There were no other significant differences between nonacquired and acquired strains.

[b] Percentages based on total number of nonacquired or acquired serotype recovered.

[c] Differences between the proportions of strains that colonize, colonize and infect, or infect were statistically analyzed for the nonacquired strains as they were also for the acquired strains. Asterisks denote the following p values: * ≤ 0.05, ** ≤ 0.01, *** ≤ 0.005, **** ≤ 0.001.

certain tendencies in regard to colonization and/or infection. The nonacquired strain of *P. aeruginosa* rarely infected lymphoma patients (13.3%, *p* 0.0478), whereas 57.1% of the serotype 7 strains that were acquired caused infection in the colonized lymphoma patient (*p* 0.0058). Also, while not significantly different, acquired strains of serotype 1 infected 46.2% of these patients without their prior colonization (*p* 0.0561), but none of the colonized patients became subsequently infected.

There were no statistical differences between the frequencies of nonacquired and acquired strains that colonized and/or infected solid tumor patients, except for those of serotype 7. Strains of this serotype that were not acquired were more likely to colonize solid tumor patients (42.9%) than were the acquired strains (5.5%, *p* 0.022). It was not unexpected that the solid tumor patient was not usually colonized solely, colonized and infected, or infected without colonization, as most strains of *P. aeruginosa* that were recovered from them either at admission or during hospitalization were, as previously mentioned, more likely to be transitory; in fact, the acquired strain rarely colonized these patients (13.3%, *p* 0.0072).

It became apparent that a serotype could show a propensity for the colonization and/or infection of a particular patient group while rarely showing the same inclination in another patient group. When considering the colonized cancer patient, it was noted that solid tumor patients were rarely colonized with nonacquired strains of serotype 1, whereas the other patient groups were. Conversely, if these strains colonized and infected the cancer patient, they were more likely to do so in leukemia or myeloma patients (*p* 0.033) or in solid tumor patients

(p 0.044) than they were to colonize and infect lymphoma patients. Acquisition of serotype 1 also influenced its behavior in that leukemia or myeloma patients who acquired strains of serotype 1 tended to become colonized and infected with them more often than did the other groups, whereas the lymphoma patient more frequently became infected without prior colonization. Colonization and infection by nonacquired strains of serotype 4 was more common in lymphoma patients than in solid tumor patients (p 0.016). Nonacquired strains of serotype 7 were more likely to colonize and infect the leukemia— myeloma patient group than they were the solid tumor patient group (p 0.44), whereas nonacquired strains of serotype 6 caused more infections without prior colonization in the latter group than they did in the former (p 0.018). Overall, colonizations alone or infections without prior colonizations by *P. aeruginosa* were no more prevalent in one group than they were in the other. However, strains of *P. aeruginosa,* whether acquired or not, were more likely to colonize and infect the leukemia–myeloma group than they were the solid tumor patient group, but not the lymphoma patient group.

Pseudomonas aeruginosa caused a total of 239 infections (51.3% of typable strains) in these cancer patients (Table 6). Repeated infections in a patient that were caused by the same serotype over time were counted as a single infection by that serotype, and multiple infections were not reflected in the total number of infections. It was apparent that acquired strains caused more infections than nonacquired strains (p 0.0012); the frequencies of infection caused by acquired strains of *P. aeruginosa* in the leukemia—myeloma, lymphoma, and solid tumor

TABLE 6. *Infections caused by P. aeruginosa in a cancer patient population*[a]

Serotype	Leukemias–myelomas		Lymphomas		Solid Tumors		Total infections	
	Not acq.	Acq.	Not acq.	Acq.	Not acq.	Acq.	Not acq.	Acq.
1	8	24***[b]	4	6	8	10	20	40***
2	8	10	1	4	3	7	12	21*
3	3	2	1	2	1	3	5	7
4	2	10*	2	3	3	4	7	17*
5	3	6	2	4	0	4	5	14*
6	5	8	4	8	5	10	14	26*
7	4	21****	4	11*	2	9*	10	41**
Totals	33	81***	18	38***	22	47****	73	166***

[a] Number of infections reflects strains that colonized and caused infections as well as those that only caused infections without prior colonization, but does not reflect multiple infections by a serotype in a patient.

[b] A two-tailed test was used to test differences between nonacquired and acquired strains. Asterisks denote the following p values: * ≤ 0.05, ** ≤ 0.01, *** ≤ 0.005, **** ≤ 0.001.

126

patient groups were 7.1% (p 0.0041), 67.9% (p 0.003), and 68.1% (p 0.001), respectively. In total infections, all serotypes when acquired, except serotype 3, caused more infections. That there is a likelihood for a specific serotype of *P. aeruginosa* to have a particular capability to cause infections after it has been acquired by a cancer patient is given credence by the significantly greater recovery of acquired serotype 7 strains from infected patients of all the cancer groups. In contrast, serotype 1, the most prevalent serotype in our hospital, when not acquired, infected approximately as many patients in the lymphoma and solid tumor groups as it did when acquired, but it had a decidedly higher incidence of infections in leukemia or myeloma patients who had acquired the serotype (p 0.0027). Serotype 4, a less commonly recovered strain in our hospital, rarely caused infections when it was part of the leukemia or myeloma patient's admission flora, but it caused a fivefold increase in infections in those patients who had acquired this organism (p 0.017).

DISCUSSION

Acquisition of *P. aeruginosa* is a common occurrence in the hospitalized cancer patient and is probably influenced by many and varied factors, such as length of hospital stay, prolonged periods of granulocytopenia, antibiotic therapy, etc. At the BCRC, patients with leukemias, myelomas, or solid tumors tend to acquire *P. aeruginosa* at higher rates than do patients with lymphoma. The serotypes most frequently acquired by solid tumor patients, a group whose immune status was the least affected of these cancer groups, reflected the prevalence and incidences of these serotypes in the BCRC patient population as well as in patients who did not have malignancies but were housed on other floors of the same hospital *(unpublished data).* This was not necessarily true of the cancer patients whose immune status was altered. Although the leukemia–myeloma group had high acquisition rates for most of the predominant serotypes, disproportionate numbers of serotypes 4 and 5 were also acquired. Conversely, serotype 1, the most prevalent strain in this hospital, was acquired by the lymphoma patient less frequently than the other serotypes, and the incidence of serotype 2 (fourth in predominance) that was acquired was significantly greater than its incidence in admission flora, whereas the acquisition frequency of the other serotypes were not.

The behavior of *P. aeruginosa* in the cancer patient appears to be based on various interrelating factors such as the underlying disease of the host, the immunological status, the antineoplastic chemotherapy, and the concurrent antibiotic therapy (4,5,8,9). That the intrinsic nature of specific serotypes can also influence the behavior of the microorganism in the host becomes apparent. It would appear that a serotype can have a higher infection potential than others. Serotype 7, whether acquired or not by the cancer patient, usually infected the patient with or without prior colonization. In contrast, acquisition of certain serotypes seems to alter the noninfecting and noncolonizing tendency that is seen in strains that are present in admission cultures. When serotype 4 was acquired by the leukemia–myeloma patient group, most of the strains caused infections and only a few strains tended to be transient, whereas strains that were present on admission were usually transitory and rarely caused infections or colonizations.

Colonization by *P. aeruginosa* commonly precedes infection caused by this organism. The incidence of strains that colonized and subsequently caused infection (bacteremias, pneumonias, abscesses, etc.) in the leukemia–myeloma patients was significantly high. On the other hand, a majority of *P. aeruginosa* strains recovered from solid tumor patients were transitory and those that did subsequently infect after colonization most frequently caused urinary tract infections.

Acquired strains caused a significantly greater number of infections than strains that were present in the patient's admission surveillance cultures. Acquired serotype 7 infected a higher percentage of patients in all groups than did the nonacquired strains. It would seem that a specific serotype of *P. aeruginosa* can be a "hospital strain," that is, predominantly found in the hospital environment. The extremely low incidence of serotype 7 in admission cultures and the extremely high acquisition rate (76.5%) in the cancer patient population seem to support this hypothesis.

Therefore, as most infections originate from the reservoir of endogenous flora and as such a large proportion of hospital-acquired infections in cancer patients are caused by *P. aeruginosa,* the importance of eliminating acquisition of this organism becomes of prime concern. Reduction in the acquisition of this bacillus alone should substantially reduce risk of early infection in the severely compromised cancer patient and thereby allow adequate time for complete antineoplastic therapy.

SUMMARY

An evaluation of the acquisition of *P. aeruginosa* serotypes by cancer patients showed that such acquisition was most frequent in the leukemia—myeloma group and that subsequent infection by the same serotype was significantly high in that group. The serotypes were acquired at rates that were generally related to their incidences in our hospital. After acquisition, certain specific serotypes were more likely to colonize and infect the various cancer patient groups, whereas others demonstrated predilection for colonization or infection. Although serotype 1 was generally the most prevalent strain in our hospital, serotype 7 colonized and infected more patients in all groups. As this serotype was seldom present in admission cultures, it could be considered a "hospital strain." Reduction in hospital acquisition of these organisms should substantially reduce the risk of early infection.

REFERENCES

1. Anderson, R. J., Schafer, L. A., Olin, D. B., and Eickhoff, T. C. (1973): Septicemia in renal transplantation recipients. *Arch. Surg.,* 106:692–694.
2. Bodey, G. P. (1970): Epidemiological studies of *Pseudomonas* species in patients with leukemia. *Am. J. Med. Sci.,* 260:82–89.
3. Burdon, D. W., and Whitby, J. L. (1967): Contamination of hospital disinfectants with *Pseudomonas* species. *Br. Med. J.,* 2:153–155.
4. Feingold, D. S. (1970): Hospital acquired infections. *N. Engl. J. Med.,* 283:1384–1391.
5. Finland, M., Jones, W. F., and Barnes, M. W. (1959): Occurrence of serious bacterial infections since the introduction of antimicrobial agents. *J.A.M.A.,* 170:2188–2197.
6. Fisher, M. W., Devlin, H. B., and Gnabasik, F. J. (1969): New immunotype schema for *Pseudomonas aeruginosa* based on protective antigens. *J. Bacteriol.,* 98:835–836.
7. Fishman, L. S., and Armstrong, D. (1972): *Pseudomonas aeruginosa* bacteremia in patients with neoplastic disease. *Cancer,* 30:764–773.

8. Frenkel, J. K. (1962): Role of corticosteroids as predisposing factors in fungal diseases. *Lab. Invest.*, 11:1192–1208.

9. Johanson, W. G., Pierce, A. K., and Sanford, J. P. (1969): Changing pharyngeal bacterial flora of hospitalized patients. *N. Engl. J. Med.*, 281:1137–1140.

10. Levine, A. S., Schimpff, S. C., Graw, R. G., Jr., and Young, R. C. (1974): Hematological malignancies and other marrow failure states: Progress in management of complicating infection. *Semin. Hematol.*, 11:141–202.

11. Lowbury, E. J. L., Thom, B. T., Lilly, H. A., Babb, J. R., and Whittall, K. (1970): Sources of *Pseudomonas aeruginosa* in patients with tracheostomy. *J. Med. Microbiol.*, 3:39–56.

12. Magarey, C. J., Chant, A. D. B., Pickford, C. R. K., and Magaray, J. R. (1971): Peritoneal drainage and systemic antibiotics after appendectomy. *Lancet*, 2:179–182.

13. Mertz, J. J., Scharer, L., and McClement, J. H. (1967): A hospital outbreak of klebsiella pneumonia from inhalation therapy with contaminated aerosol solutions. *Am. Rev. Resp. Dis.*, 95:454–460.

14. Moffet, H. L., Allan, D., and Williams, T. (1967): Bacteria recovered from distilled water and inhalation therapy equipment. *Am. J. Dis. Child.*, 114:13–20.

15. Moody, M. R., Young, V. M., Kenton, D. M., and Vermeulen, G. D. (1972): *Pseudomonas aeruginosa* in a center for cancer research: Distribution of intraspecies types from human and environmental sources. *J. Infect. Dis.*, 125:95–101.

16. Price, D. J. E., and Sleigh, J. D. (1970): Control of infection due to *Klebsiella aerogenes* in a neurosurgical unit by withdrawal of all antibiotics. *Lancet*, 2:1213–1215.

17. Pruitt, B. A., Jr., Flemma, R. J., DeVincenti, F. C., Foley, F. D., and Mason, A. D., Jr. (1970): Pulmonary complications in burn patients: A comparative study of 697 patients. *J. Thorac. Cardiovasc. Surg.*, 59:7–20.

18. Schimpff, S. C., Moody, M. R., and Young, V. M. (1970): Relationship of colonization with *Pseudomonas aeruginosa* to development of Pseudomonas bacteremia in cancer patients. In: *Antimicrob. Agents and Chemother., 1969*, pp. 240–244, American Society of Microbiology, Bethesda, Md.

19. Schimpff, S. C., Satterlee, W., Young, V. M., and Serpick, A. (1971): Empiric therapy with carbenicillin and gentamicin for febrile patients with cancer and granulocytopenia. *N. Engl. J. Med.*, 284:1061–1065.

20. Schimpff, S. C., Young, V. M., Greene, W. H., Vermuelen, G. D., Moody, M. R., and Wiernik, P. H. (1972): Origin of infection in acute nonlymphocytic leukemia. Significance of hospital acquisition of potential pathogens. *Ann. Intern. Med.,* 77:707–714.

21. Schimpff, S. C., Greene, W. H., Young, V. M., and Wiernik, P. H. (1973): *Pseudomonas* septicemia: Incidence, epidemiology, prevention and therapy in patients with advanced cancer. *Eur. J. Cancer,* 9:449–455.

22. Schimpff, S. C., Miller, R. M., Polakavetz, S., and Hornick, R. B. (1974): Infection in the severely traumatized patient. *Ann. Surg.,* 179:352–357.

23. Selden, R., Lee, S., Wang, W. L., Bennett, J. V., and Eickhoff, T. C. (1971): Nosocomial Klebsiella infections: Intestinal colonization as a reservoir. *Ann. Intern. Med.,* 74:657–664.

24. Sickles, E. A., Young, V. M., Greene, W. H., and Wiernik, P. H. (1973): Pneumonia in acute leukemia. *Ann. Intern. Med.,* 79:528–534.

25. Young, V. M., and Moody, M. R. (1974): Serotyping of *Pseudomonas aeruginosa. J. Infect. Dis.,* 130:S47–S52.

Subject Index

A

Acidity, gastric, and colonization by *Pseudomonas,* 99

Aerators, and prevention of contamination in sinks, 89

African violet plants and soil, *Pseudomonas* in, 9, 12, 14, 15

Agricultural areas, *Pseudomonas* in, 1-24. *See also* Plants; Soil

Antibiotics
and gastrointestinal colonization of *Pseudomonas,* 71-73, 98, 101
resistance or susceptibility of *Pseudomonas* to, 15, 39-43

Artichokes, *Pseudomonas* in, 10

Aster beds, *Pseudomonas* in, 9

Azalea plants and soil, *Pseudomonas* in, 9, 12, 14

B

Bacterial interference, and gastrointestinal colonization of *Pseudomonas,* 101-102

Baths, as source of *Pseudomonas* in hospitals, 80
in whirlpool baths, 61, 84

Bean plants, *Pseudomonas* colonization in, 15, 17-19

Beet plants and soil, *Pseudomonas* in, 10, 14

Begonia beds, *Pseudomonas* in, 9

Broccoli, *Pseudomonas* in, 10

Brussel sprouts, *Pseudomonas* pathogenicity in, 17-19

Burn patients, 59-73
control program for, 60-61
food for
cultures of samples of, 64-65
and dietary control of *Pseudomonas* infections, 70-73
gastrointestinal colonization of *Pseudomonas* in, 62-63, 78
antibiotics affecting, 71-73
hospital acquisition of *Pseudomonas* in, 62-63, 78
in hyperendemic situation, 60
primary wound sepsis in, 62
and transmission of *Pseudomonas,* 77-93

C

Cabbage, *Pseudomonas* in, 10, 68

Cancer patients, and *Pseudomonas* acquisition in hospitals, 111-129
colonization and infection with, 121-127
detection of, 113-114
incidence of, 114-118
serotypes in, 116, 119, 121, 128, 129
transitory strains in, 118-121

Carbenicillin, resistance to, 15, 39, 40, 42, 43-44